IMMUNIZATION

IMMUNIZATION
How Vaccines Became Controversial

Stuart Blume

REAKTION BOOKS

Published by Reaktion Books Ltd
Unit 32, Waterside
44–48 Wharf Road
London N1 7UX, UK
www.reaktionbooks.co.uk

First published 2017
Copyright © Stuart Blume 2017

Printed and bound in Great Britain
by TJ International, Padstow, Cornwall

A catalogue record for this book is available from the British Library

ISBN 978 1 78023 837 1

CONTENTS

ONE

WHAT DO VACCINES DO?

Hope

If its films are any kind of guide, the English-speaking world views the prospect of a pandemic with the fascination of a trapped man watching an approaching snake. There is a sense of horror, of inevitability. Films about epidemics show us people in their thousands (or more) dropping in the streets, social disintegration and approaching havoc. However, there is a catharsis. In many of these films there are heroes or heroines, doctors or scientists, who ultimately save what is left of the human race. Some of these movies, such as John Ford's 1931 film of Sinclair Lewis's novel *Arrowsmith*, were made long ago, but most are fairly recent. Think of the 1995 film *Outbreak*, starring Dustin Hoffman and Morgan Freeman. Or the 2007 film *I Am Legend*, starring Will Smith. Or the popular TV series *The Last Ship*. Or Steven Soderbergh's gripping 2011 version, *Contagion*. Soderbergh's film opens with an American business executive, Beth Emhoff, taken ill on her way home from Hong Kong. She's coughing and sweating. We see others similarly affected, in Hong Kong, London, Tokyo . . . This is turning into a public health emergency though it is totally unclear how it started, or where, or what is causing it. It is a private tragedy as well. Of course it is many private tragedies, but the film focuses on how Beth's collapse and rapid death affect her family. Her husband Mitch is at first incredulous, then bereft, then put into an isolation ward, and finally discovered to be immune. The public health side of things focuses on the Center for Disease Control (CDC) based in Atlanta, Georgia, and in particular on an epidemiologist named Erin Mears who has to trace and map the spread of the disease, on her boss Ellis Cheever, and on Ally Hexhall, a virologist who'll be given the job of identifying the causal agent, which proves to be a virus. The action shifts to Geneva, where the World Health Organization (WHO) is based, and where reports are coming in of deaths and millions of cases from some of the world's most densely populated metropolises. The WHO, which has developed protocols for dealing with this kind of emergency, is going to send Dr Leonora Orontes to investigate. What precautionary measures should governments be advised to take? Should schools be closed? Is there a risk of panicking people needlessly? How does the virus spread? Epidemiological investigation would have to establish how infectious it is. What kind of virus is it? Is there a chance that a known pathogen (anthrax? smallpox? 'Bird flu'?) has been turned into a weapon and that this epidemic has been started deliberately?

It's the work of epidemiologist Mears (out in the field) and of the virologists manipulating samples in their laboratories that forms the core of the movie. Because Mears is able to establish that Beth was 'patient number 1', and that she became sick as a result of eating some infected poultry, and because the virologists succeed in identifying and then growing the virus, a vaccine can be made and mankind saved. But this isn't a documentary, so it's embellished by a number of dramatic flourishes, some of which point neatly to real-life complications, dilemmas and concerns. Orontes, who is dispatched to Hong Kong, suspects that that is where it all started, but discovers that the authorities are anxious to prevent any such announcement being made. Moreover, plenty of people think there is money to be made. We are introduced to Alan Krumwiede, an influential (but shady) blogger, who claims that there's a simple, cheap 'natural' cure for the disease, which the public health 'establishment' and the pharmaceutical industry are keeping secret. They want to develop and profit from an expensive vaccine. We subsequently learn that he is hoping to make money himself from this plant extract. Demand becomes insatiable, and riots break out at drugstores across the USA as people try to get hold of it. There are roadblocks and looting. The impression we are given is that the social disruption caused by the epidemic is at least as serious, and certainly as frightening, as the virus. An epidemiology of fear is evoked. As one of the characters points out, in order to get sick you have to be in contact with an infected person or something that they've touched. In order to get scared you just have to get in contact with TV or the Internet.

If this dramatic rendering is compared with the histories of real epidemics – comparisons that characters in the movie often make – it is clear that the film-makers did a great deal of preparatory research. (I wasn't surprised to be told that that they'd visited the World Health Organization to learn how epidemics are dealt with.) Though the likelihood of an epidemic leading to social breakdown surely varies from one society to another, a documentary about a real-life global epidemic could draw on this account of a fictional one. It is not just that the story is a distillation from real-life happenings. It is also that it provides a script: a resource for writing about epidemics. Nearly thirty years ago the eminent historian of medicine Charles Rosenberg offered a dramaturgical way of writing about epidemics.[1] Inspired by Albert Camus' novel *The Plague* (1947), Rosenberg suggests that in the past epidemics tended to evolve in a well-structured narrative sequence. Act I of the imaginary play is a community's reluctant acceptance and public acknowledgement that disease has struck. Act II, which he calls 'Managing Randomness', involves the search for some explanatory framework: a way of making sense of the fact that some die while others survive. It is this framework that can provide a guide to action and to control. In earlier times this framework tended to be rooted in widely held assumptions about proper and responsible behaviour. Then, in Act III, a 'public response' is negotiated: a set of 'collective rites integrating cognitive and emotional elements'. Whether these rites emphasize collective fasting and prayer, or quarantine, they represent an enactment of community solidarity. Finally, in the last act of Charles Rosenberg's narrative, the number of cases has declined. The epidemic is under control. Some have died and others have recovered. Now there is time for remembering and reflecting, though this can probably be entrusted to the historians. 'Has a heedless society reverted to its accustomed ways of doing things as soon as denial became once more a plausible option?' 'Epidemics', Rosenberg notes, 'have always provided occasion for retrospective moral judgment'.[2] If this was a reflection on an era when there were no virologists, written for an age when time and space hadn't been compressed to the extent they are today, then *Contagion* provides us with an update. It offers a way of imagining and writing about epidemics as they evolve, as they spread, and as the desperate search for control – today centred more on the laboratory than on the house of prayer – gathers pace.

Fear

When we are told that some horrific pandemic is in prospect – something like the 1918 Spanish flu that killed tens of millions of people (an estimated 3 to 5 per cent of the world's population), or that a previously unknown virus has emerged from its remote jungle home (as in *Contagion*) – we now turn expectantly to virologists like Ally Hexhall and the high-security labs in which they go about their business. An example that hit the news in the first weeks of 2016, and that almost no one who wasn't a virologist had heard of up till then, is the Zika virus. It was discovered in the Zika forest, in Uganda, by researchers who were actually investigating yellow fever. Both viruses, and that responsible for dengue, are spread by the same species of mosquito, *Aedes aegypti*. Infection with the Zika virus was nothing to panic about. Although the virus had been found in 1947, the first reported case of someone becoming sick from it was only in 1964. After three days of fever and some aches and pains, the victim had fully recovered. Studies showed that many cases of infection were totally without symptoms. But as the virus was carried further afield its effects appeared to change. Epidemics in various Pacific islands in the early 2000s showed more serious symptoms, in particular Guillain-Barré syndrome. And then it found its way to Central and South America. Evidence began to accumulate that if a pregnant woman became infected her baby might be born with an abnormally small head (a condition known as microcephaly). A significantly higher than usual number of babies have been born with microcephaly in Brazil, where the virus has spread rapidly. Researchers are discovering that it is not only mosquitoes that spread it. Some women seem to have picked it up from infected semen and possibly even from sweat. Work on developing a vaccine is under way: in Brazil's Butantan Institute; in the u.s. National Institute of Health; in pharmaceutical giants like GSK and Sanofi Pasteur; and in some small biotechnology companies. Estimates as to when it might become available differ enormously. Of course it is not as though nothing is being done while the vaccine is being developed. While the scientists are working, something has to be done to help people who are affected (there is no anti-Zika drug yet) and also to limit the spread of the contagion. Simple measures like covering barrels of drinking water can help. Restricting people's movements, especially people who might be infected, has been used for centuries to limit the spread of infectious disease. Now there are new and more sophisticated ways of identifying people who might be infected. That is why, a few years ago, many airports installed thermal scanners. They were intended to identify passengers whose raised body temperature indicated possible 'swine flu'.

Writing in 1986, as the world was struggling to come to terms with the start of the AIDS epidemic, Roy Porter, Britain's pre-eminent historian of medicine until his death in 2002, wrote:

> What's dangerous about fear, however, is that it rarely comes neat, but is always manipulated and exploited. As a consequence, its objects become displaced and its functions perverted . . . The Black Death, for instance, was said to be the doing of the Jews (who were massacred all across Europe for their alleged responsibility) . . . And later, in the 19th century, the new, terrifying cholera pandemics were similarly exploited to exacerbate social alarm. Arising from the degraded depths of Asia and then, when sweeping across Europe striking down the lumpenproletarian scum, cholera was, in the eyes of many official spokesmen, nature's way of demonstrating that the great unwashed were intrinsically polluted, and diseased.[3]

Without questioning the seriousness of the disease, Porter was concerned that fear of the AIDS epidemic was being whipped up because media moguls were convinced that 'fear sells newspapers'. Keeping out people who are different from ourselves, especially when they are suspected of carrying disease, still has great emotive, and thus political, force. While there is much to be said for restricting the movement of infectious individuals, the emotive appeal of quarantine easily spills over into generalized fear of groups that are thought to be not only susceptible but also carriers of infection. For example, at the start of the AIDS epidemic in the U.S. in 1981, immigrants from Haiti appeared particularly numerous among those affected, resulting in stigmatization and exclusion of people from Haiti, sick or not.

The dramatizations of a pandemic in a movie like *Contagion* and the forecasts produced by virologists and by the pharmaceutical industry feed into and off one another. The movies are based on a reading of previous epidemics, but at the same time they provide a discursive resource – a kind of plot – for virologists thinking and writing about the future. Nathan Wolfe's *The Viral Storm: The Dawn of a New Pandemic Age* was published by Penguin books in 2011, the same year that the movie *Contagion* was released. Wolfe, who is a virologist, suggests that the term 'pandemic' should be used to describe the spread of a virus from a few people to many people in many places, and quite irrespective of its deadliness. 'In fact, from my perspective,' he writes, 'it's possible we could have a pandemic and not even notice it.'[4] If a handful of people were infected with a virus that produced no symptoms of illness, and if those people were distributed over the various regions of the world, then this would constitute a pandemic. While far from the imagery of the pandemic disaster movie, from the perspective of *The Viral Storm* any virus is a *potential* source of danger. There is a great deal in the book about the deficient animal husbandry and butchering practices that give rise to new viral threats. The hunting and butchering of wild animals, the mingling of household pets and animals intended for human consumption, and intensive animal farming: all of these practices influence the likelihood that a virus to which its animal host had adapted will enter a human population with potentially disastrous consequences. And of course the growing interconnectedness of people everywhere, thanks to modern means of transportation, offers the virus vast intercontinental possibilities. Wolfe tells us that a collaborator of his had examined the rate at which new viruses had been identified over the past century. That study suggests that in the coming decade an average of at least one or two new viruses per year are likely to be found: a result of growing mobility, lifestyle changes and increasingly sophisticated virus-hunting. Wolfe, like a number of other authors, leaves us in no doubt that future influenza and possibly other pandemics are inevitable. As director of 'Global Viral Forecasting', he wants to convince his readers that pandemics don't occur randomly, and that with the right surveillance tools they can be predicted – and prevented. 'Prediction and prevention of pandemics will not be easy, but there is much we can do right now, and the advances that are steadily occurring will allow us to do even more in the future.'[5] A study published in the same year by researchers at the European Centre for Disease Prevention and Control proceeds along similar lines.[6] Previous work had suggested that hundreds of human pathogens had emerged or re-emerged over the previous half century. These authors set out to identify plausible threats facing Europe in 2020 'on the basis of current knowledge about disease as well as about changing social-ecological contexts'. All of their scenarios make depressing reading.

As in most of the pandemic disaster movies – and hopefully without the almost complete destruction of the human race that some display – mankind will be able to ride the storm, at least if provided with comprehensive surveillance using the very latest computer and information technology, and given sufficient investment in vaccine development. Of course, how far all this technology, or the best efforts of virologists and the pharmaceutical industry, can help human communities deal with the panic and social disintegration displayed in the movies, is a separate issue. Could it be that epidemic preparedness requires something in addition to the ability to rapidly produce a new vaccine? Certainly, fears of bioterrorism have provoked calls in the United States for emergency powers that would legalize the involuntary sequestering and examination of suspects – not suspected terrorists, but people merely suspected of having been infected by one or other 'weaponized' pathogen.

If the havoc wrought on a community depends on how its members respond, then a movie like *Contagion* does more than entertain. Watching a movie like this should not only reinforce our trust in the white-coated virologists, but it should also enable us mentally to rehearse how we'd behave. Will we trust what government representatives, the CDC people in the movie, have to say when they explain the risks they believe we face?

Immunity

What do we hope for from the scientists? What exactly is it that *Contagion*'s scientists are trying to develop? Wikipedia gives us a nice simple definition of what a vaccine is: 'A vaccine is a biological preparation that provides active acquired immunity to a particular disease.' That helps somewhat. It is biological – made from something found in nature – and it is connected to a particular disease. So it is not like a tonic or an aspirin. But what is particular about what a vaccine does? What is 'active acquired immunity'?

Many kinds of microscopically small organisms potentially threaten the human body. Our planet is inhabited by far greater numbers of viruses, bacteria, parasites and fungi than of any other kind of living organism. They are not all bad. We humans coexist quite happily with some of them. Indeed some of the bacteria that live in our guts, stomachs and genitalia actually help us avoid infection, or they help us digest the food we consume. All the foreign microorganisms in the human body, whether helpful or harmful, display distinctive markers which the immune system can recognize. If a harmful invader is signalled, then the immune system has the job of destroying it. A vaccine is a substance that helps it do so. Vaccines usually contain antigens, which are bits of the disease-causing organism, which stimulate the body's immune system to fight off a potential infection. The vaccine helps the immune system to recognize the pathogen and to launch the right kind of counter-attack before the sickness has taken hold.

Vaccines help my body's immune system protect me against infection. If we go on to ask *how* they do that, things get complicated. This is not only because the immune system has a range of defensive weapons at its disposal, but also because the science of how it works, immunology, is rapidly advancing. There is a special circulatory system that carries 'lymph', a transparent fluid containing lymphocytes, around the body. The lymphocytes are crucial participants in the body's defences. There are B cells, which grow in bone marrow, and T cells, which mature in the thymus, up in the chest. A useful document produced by the American National Institutes of Health explains that the B and T cells have somewhat different functions and are responsible for distinct forms of immunity.[7] B cells produce antibodies that circulate in blood and the lymph streams and attach to foreign antigens to mark them for destruction by other immune cells. B cells are part of what is known as antibody-mediated immunity. B cells have a range of functions, one of which is overall coordination and regulation of the body's immune response. There are also T cells that, like the B cells, patrol the blood and lymph. But these T cells can do more than recognize a foreign invader; they can also attack and destroy cells that they recognize as foreign. T cells are responsible for what is known as 'cell-mediated immunity'. Some of the T cells are there to prod B cells into making antibodies, as well as activating other T cells and immune system scavenger cells called macrophages. There are T cells which can turn into killer cells that attack and destroy infected cells, as well as circulating scavenger cells known as phagocytes, which have the job of engulfing an unwelcome microbe. And crucially, there are also memory cells. When the army of B and T cells begins its work of defending the body it transforms some of its members into what are called memory cells. After the defence has been successfully mounted and the infection beaten off, the army is 'demobilized'. But the memory cells remain on alert, and are able to recognize the same invading pathogen if and when it returns. Thanks to this warning, the immune system can swing rapidly into action, so that the body is better prepared than it was the first time. This is the process known as naturally acquired immunity, and most human beings benefit from it from the earliest days of life. Indeed certain types of immune cells are actually passed from mother to foetus in the course of a normal pregnancy. Newborn babies generally enter the world with temporary immunity to certain diseases.

Distinguishable from this naturally acquired immunity is so-called artificially acquired immunity. As its name suggests this results from something introduced into the body, such as a vaccine. A distinction is also made (and unlike much of the above this has been known for almost a century) between active and passive acquired immunity. Artificially acquired passive immunity results when antibodies produced by another animal or human are given to someone to prevent or treat disease. For example, administering tetanus antitoxin or rabies immunoglobulin to someone is a way of conferring passive immunity. This type of immunization works rapidly, but protection only lasts for a short time. So today its main use is for short-term protection of people when they are particularly vulnerable, such as immediately after exposure to a serious disease. Vaccines are intended to provide active immunity: that is, to stimulate the immune system into mounting its defences.

Some of the characters in *Contagion* must know all this. The virologists, struggling in their laboratories to isolate the virus and make a vaccine from it, know all about how vaccines work. This kind of knowledge is essential to what they do. For the public health professionals at the CDC and WHO it's different. Their expertise is in understanding the dynamics of an epidemic, in establishing the ways in which and the speed at which it spreads. Their responsibility is to map out a strategy for gathering samples, for containing the outbreak in so far as is possible, and for deployment of the vaccine when it comes. The laypeople in the movie, like most of us, know almost nothing of virology, immunology or epidemiology.

Now we can start to see that, however necessary they are, there is something important that definitions (such as the Wikipedia definition of a vaccine) cannot do. They cannot throw light on the variety of meanings that people attach to 'things' (in the widest possible sense of the word). Artefacts of any kind mean different things to people involved with them in different ways. If we want to understand why a particular group uses a particular object in one way, while another group uses it in another way, then the dictionary definition is of little help. An example can help make the point more clearly. Think of an aircraft. Though vitally important for all those involved, an aircraft obviously means something different to the engineer employed to put its engine together, the pilot whose responsibility it is to fly hundreds of people safely from one end of the earth to the other, and to the businessman commuting weekly between Amsterdam and London. We can add to the list almost endlessly. There are the cleaners who swarm aboard after the passengers have disembarked, the baggage handlers, the people whose sleep is disturbed by aircraft noise. So it is with the vaccine in *Contagion*: a daily struggle in the laboratory for one, an essential tool for another, and a last hope for a third.

For biomedical scientists, vaccines are substances that produce a certain kind of effect on the body. For them, a key number in thinking about how effective a vaccine is is the percentage of 'seroconversion'. How effective is the vaccine in stimulating the body to develop detectable antibodies to the pathogen in question? It takes time for the immune system to be prodded into action. But after extensive seroconversion has taken place, the person will test positive for the presence of antibodies to a specific bacterium or virus. When public health professionals or international health bureaucrats or ministers of health think about using a vaccine on a large scale, they will be more concerned with different kinds of numbers. By how much will vaccination reduce deaths or serious illness? And increasingly, what will it cost?

Protecting the Community

For professionals struggling at the front line of public health, establishing the precise nature of a vaccine-induced immune response is much less important than establishing how the vaccine can best be used. The first vaccines were developed and used long before anyone knew about antibodies, let alone viruses or T cells. It is the epidemiologists and public health professionals who are expected to develop an appropriate vaccination strategy. How many shots are required for effective protection? At what ages is each best given? If it is given too early the vaccine might interfere with maternal antibodies protecting a newborn baby, or the effect might wear off before the time of maximum risk. If it is given too late children may have already been infected.

Though vaccination isn't the only tool used in protecting the health of communities, it has become an increasingly important one. Vaccination schedules are becoming more and more complex as one new vaccine after another is added. Many of the vaccines routinely offered to children today are quite new. For example, in the USA varicella (chickenpox) vaccine has been recommended since 1996, vaccination against hepatitis A since 2000, and pneumococcal vaccine since 2001. In September 2015 the UK began to provide the vaccine against meningitis B to two-month-old babies. A child today will be immunized against many more diseases than its parents, and probably twice as many as its grandparents. The result of these additions, and of reformulations of old vaccines in more expensive forms, is that the cost of childhood vaccination is constantly rising. Doctors without Borders points out that while children in poor countries are now vaccinated against twice as many diseases as in 2000, the cost of the vaccines has risen 68-fold.[8] In England and Wales the immunization schedule now prescribes that a child will have received fourteen different antigens between the ages of two months and fourteen years. It is approximately the same in Australia and the USA. This doesn't mean fourteen injections. Some of the antigens (such as diphtheria, tetanus and whooping cough, or measles, mumps and rubella) are combined in one shot, while most need to be given two or three times to ensure long-term protection. Some aren't injected but are given as drops or a nasal spray. Vaccination schedules aren't the same everywhere. A Dutch child will receive eleven antigens, starting at the age of six to nine weeks, while an Indian child is recommended to receive three at birth and another nine by the time it celebrates its first birthday.

Not all parents actually turn up with their child at the appointed time and place, though in the industrialized world most do. There is a lot of concern about those who don't, however, and about the fact that their numbers seem to be rising. This matters because when the vast majority of people are immune, a pathogen (a bacterium or virus) has so few receptive hosts to infect that its transmission is blocked. This phenomenon, known as 'herd immunity', means that even the few people who aren't vaccinated are unlikely to become infected. One reason (but not the only one) why 'coverage rates' get so much attention is that herd immunity only occurs when they are very high – typically around 80–90 per cent of a population having been vaccinated. The exact number at which herd immunity kicks in cannot be given. It varies, depending on the effectiveness of the vaccine. It also depends on how infectious a particular pathogen is: something that the epidemiologists in *Contagion* were anxious to establish with some urgency. They have a number for talking about this: the parameter known as R_0. This parameter gives the average number of people likely to be infected by someone who is already infected, in an otherwise unaffected population. The higher the number, the more contagious the disease. Thus the R_0 for HIV/AIDS is two to five, for polio five to seven, and for measles fifteen to eighteen.

In much of Asia and Africa, vaccination rates are only starting to approach those crucial 80–90 per cent rates, and then for only a few basic vaccines. The World Health Organization's website tells us that globally in 2014, 86 per cent of children had received three doses of polio vaccine and 85 per cent had received one dose of measles vaccine. But numbers like these are enormously influenced by data from very populous countries such as China, India and Brazil. Small countries with very low coverage don't have much effect on these global numbers. Nor of course do regional or socio-economic inequalities appear in these global figures, though in some countries (including India) they are very large indeed.

Although it is extremely difficult to distinguish the effects of vaccination from those of improved living conditions (hygiene, nutrition, water quality) and of improved maternal and neonatal care, there is no doubt that vaccination has contributed vastly to reducing death and serious disease among children. For example, polio cases have decreased by over 99 per cent since 1988, from an estimated 350,000 cases then, to 359 reported cases in 2014. In 1955 there were 29,000 cases of polio in the USA alone, and 1,000 deaths, but there have been no cases at all since the late 1960s. Global measles deaths have decreased by 79 per cent from an estimated 546,800 in 2000 to 114,900 in 2014. Because there are many regions of the world in which coverage is far too low, so that many children are still becoming sick or dying, for the last forty years considerable effort has been devoted to extending the reach of vaccination programmes, as well as the number of antigens being provided to children in poor countries.

Few parents taking their child to be vaccinated know or care much about these things, and nor do many older people going for their annual flu jab. Most of us don't know much about the immune system or R_0 and not many of us know much about measles, polio or malaria mortality statistics. So why do most parents, at least those who have ready access to vaccination services, take their children to be vaccinated? Is it a passive response, simply what most other parents do and what seems to be expected? Or does it involve a more active assessment of the kinds of risks the child seems likely to face? Not all the risks of course. There are all too many parents whose children face daily risks of violence, homelessness or hunger. These parents have to develop multifaceted strategies to try to ensure their children's survival. We need a more limited focus. What health risks do children face, and what risks do their parents think they face? The risks of catching an infection as estimated by epidemiologists will not necessarily correspond with parents' sense of the risks they think their children face. We are becoming more and more sensitive to risks, and increasingly risk-averse, with the result that parents' views about vaccination may well be neither consistent nor stable over time.

Goods and Bads, Rights and Wrongs

Vaccines have long figured in two different understandings of health. They help protect the vulnerable body of the individual child. And they protect the 'social body', the community. The concept of herd immunity links the two. In the era of globalization in which we now live, a new dimension, the global, has been added. Claiming that health, or maybe immunization as a route to health, is a 'global public good', is to claim first that it's a 'good'. Of course 'goods' are the things we acquire or buy (clothes, apples, books) and the services we make use of. But the word also has another meaning (the opposite of 'bads'). Most of the goods we consume are 'private'. We pay for our daily bread or rice, and once we've eaten it, that's it. It's gone. By contrast, 'public goods' (such as fresh air, city parks or public libraries) are available to anyone, with no need to pay. They don't get used up, and nor does my making use of them mean that there is less available for you. Global public goods are then defined as public goods the benefits from which are available across national borders, globally. Anyone anywhere, irrespective of ability to pay, can enjoy the benefits. There is no commercial incentive to produce goods of this kind. Since by definition they are available to all irrespective of ability to pay there is no apparent profit to be made. That is why at the national level governments step in to underwrite the costs of social services, drinking water, roads, basic research and education . . . or at least they used to. The argument has then been made that, since no national government has a responsibility to pay for *global* public goods, some other kind of inter- or trans-national entity has to do so.

The anthropologist Veena Das has suggested that because it meets all these criteria immunization is a clear example of a global public good. More importantly, she explains, it is being treated as such. What does this imply? That resources are being deployed, vaccination campaigns financed, with the notion of *global* benefit principally in mind. This implies that priority is attached neither to the health needs of the individual child nor to those of the community it lives in, but to some notion of all the people in the world. What might prioritizing 'the global' mean in practice? Drawing on research she carried out in the Indian state of Madhya Pradesh in 1997, Das illustrates what it might mean. She tells us of an obviously very sick baby she came across in a tiny and impoverished rural hamlet. No one there had any food. The women were waiting, hoping that the men of the village would soon return after managing to earn some rice. Concerned about the feverish baby's condition, she asked if the women knew about oral rehydration therapy. 'They did not know anything about it – the ANM [a state employed nurse-midwife] never came up to the hamlet. However, on National Immunization Day last year they had all been taken to the school in the main hamlet and the babies were administered the oral polio vaccine drops.'[9] Struggling for existence, at the very margin of sustainable life, it is hard to imagine that polio vaccination was a health priority for people there.

Why do millions of rural mothers like these trudge long distances to have their baby vaccinated, maybe even foregoing a day's income to do so? Is it because they are convinced that getting their baby vaccinated against hepatitis B or rotavirus is essential to its future health and well-being, even though they have probably never heard of these diseases? Is it because the health visitor who comes to their village from time to time persuades them? Or because other mothers in the village do so? Or is it because they are compelled by the promise or denial of something they value? Veena Das quotes a public health official claiming credit for having devised the strategy of denying birth certificates – and thus the welfare payments that go with them – to babies who had not been immunized. She suggests, to my mind correctly, that such a measure 'signals an arrogance on the part of international organizations that can deny rights to citizens in the pursuit of aims and targets that are no doubt important' but which aren't necessarily the highest good from the perspective of ordinary people.[10] Families denied child welfare payments as a result of non-vaccination are likely to be precisely those whose need is greatest. Though this essay is based on research carried out in India, the issues it raises are universal. Thinking about why most British, or Canadian, or Italian parents take their babies to be vaccinated, we can ask the same questions. Is it because they have become convinced of the health benefit of immunization? Or because their family doctor advises it? Or because other mothers in their social circle do so? Or is it because, as in some countries, they are compelled to do so by government sanctions?

Children in the United States need to be able to show that they have been fully immunized before they can enter a state school. The same is true of some Canadian provinces. In Australia there's no compulsion but parents are denied certain welfare payments if their child is not fully vaccinated. The position in European countries varies considerably. About half of them have no compulsory vaccinations, while the others have one or more, most commonly polio, though in a few countries diphtheria and tetanus or hepatitis B vaccinations are mandatory. Irrespective of whether it is mandatory or voluntary, vaccination rates in Western European countries are generally high. Is that all that matters? As long as parents take their children to be vaccinated, does it make any difference whether they do so because they are trying to protect their child, or out of altruism (in the interest of the community as a whole), or because they are compelled? Focusing only on numbers, especially coverage rates, implies that it does not really matter what lies behind the numbers. It might suggest that faced with a population so recalcitrant that an acceptable rate of vaccination can only be achieved by compulsion or coercion then so be it. The end justifies the means. But does it?

In recent years a number of arguments against vaccination built on coercion have been developed. One is pragmatic. As historian Paul Greenough explains, in a classic analysis of coercive smallpox vaccination practices in South Asia,

> coercion can leave behind a residue of resentment that sours public attitudes toward the next vaccination campaign. The social memory of traumatic encounters with the state and its agents runs deep in South Asia, where low literacy levels paradoxically require that public *events* be kept in consciousness through oral accounts and rumors rather than by written means. Rumors that disparage the motives or revile the conduct of government agents are as great an enemy of public health as the disease because they lead to avoidance and opposition.[11]

Writing in 1995, Greenough also touched on a quite different argument, of a kind that was of growing importance at the time. How could vaccinating people by force be justifiable in Bangladesh when it would be more or less inconceivable in Berlin, Birmingham or Boston? In the last few years there has been growing attention (if not universal respect) for human rights, for individual rights, for citizens' rights. In particular, and hastened by responses to the AIDS crisis in the 1980s, the ethical issues involved have been highlighted and debated. What kind of threats justify what kind of compulsions on the part of governments? If 85 per cent of children are immunized, is it right for the state to demand it of the remaining 15 per cent, even those who might have doubts or objections? Should there be 'opt-out' clauses on the grounds of belief or conscience, as there are in some places? A few years ago, Italian policymakers removed the element of compulsion, and left it to individual regions with a good overall immunization coverage to let parents decide for themselves.

On the other hand, a growing sense of threat may push politicians in the other direction. Since January 2016 parents in the state of California no longer have the right to claim exemption from vaccination on any other grounds than medical. Perhaps provoked by the implications of this same sense of threat, ethicists have begun to reflect on various other vaccine-related dilemmas. When an epidemic is coming, and although there is a vaccine it is still in short supply, who should have priority? Those at greatest risk (for example the family members of people already infected)? Healthcare workers (since they can do the most good when healthy)? Children? The fragile elderly who are most likely to succumb if infected? Another issue concerns the targeting of risk groups. Epidemiologists may identify a particular group (whether based on ethnicity, sexual preferences, age and gender and so on) who are at greater than average risk of being infected. Is it reasonable to vaccinate members of this group alone, as many countries did when a costly new hepatitis B vaccine became available? Or could this be regarded as stigmatizing and discriminatory in the same way as restricting their freedom of movement or forbidding them from donating blood?

Doubt

What do parents think about the vaccination of their child? Obviously it is hard to generalize, since the social, cultural and environmental worlds which families inhabit differ so greatly. Where a child's health is constantly challenged by different kinds of mosquitoes, by lack of clean drinking water, by inadequate nutrition, demand for the protection conferred by vaccination can exceed what an under-resourced health system can provide. But then again, lack of access to that health system, or religious beliefs, may reduce this demand. In the industrialized world most parents take vaccination pretty much for granted most of the time. We take our child along to the doctor, or the child welfare clinic, where it is given the scheduled shots together with checks on its growth and development. In

Western Europe, North America and many other places this is now normal parental behaviour. As I said before, maybe we do it out of conviction (it seems a good and easy way of protecting little Johnny or little Lisa against measles, or whooping cough, or hepatitis B). Or maybe we do it because the doctor, or the nurse, or the health visitor, whom we trust, advises us to. Most of us don't think too hard about why we have our child vaccinated. Most parents quietly wait their turn. But things change and views are destabilized when we believe that we are faced by an epidemic of some new killer virus. As schools are closed, or we are told not to travel or even shake hands, or are advised not to become pregnant, normal life is disrupted. Comparisons with the 1918 Spanish flu epidemic, or forecasts of the number of people likely to become infected, add to people's anxiety. As the prospect of a vaccine comes to seem our best or only hope, vaccination is no longer just something we do. The heightened expectations that come into play lead us to draw on a different cultural repertoire. We remember the movies we have seen, and the fact that in them it is the scientists who save us. We want vaccine and we want it now!

To suggest that in thinking about vaccination, parents veer between passive acceptance and demand verging on panic, does not capture the whole situation. There is a third position, a more sceptical one, which comes in stronger and weaker versions. Some parents reject vaccination completely. Some of them are convinced that a child's immunity must be built up 'naturally', rather than being 'enhanced' with what they see as pathogenic material. They organize 'chickenpox parties' or find other ways of letting a sick child infect theirs. Some parents are convinced that vaccines lead to various diseases, of which the causes are often unclear, such as autism, narcolepsy or irritable bowel syndrome. Though in the industrialized world there are not many such parents, they are said to be disproportionately visible on the Internet. The weak version – a sense of doubt, of uncertainty – is more widespread, though it doesn't really lend itself either to star-studded dramatization or even to massive online visibility. In the final chapter of this book I will discuss what I believe to be the sources of this uncertainty, and why I think it is spreading.

Eula Biss, a writer who teaches in the English department of a leading u.s. university, has produced an evocative account of her own reflections. She writes of the urge to protect the baby she was expecting, an urge that she felt powerfully, and which led her to look into how she could best do so. She started reading about immunization before her baby was born, and soon ran into a mountain of debates regarding the safety and efficacy of the various vaccines, and disputes surrounding the additives and preservatives – formaldehyde, mercury, aluminium – that they often contain. Her book is a meditation on the notion of immunity, on the cultural significance of blood and the vampire myth, on the deeply entrenched notion of the culturally 'Other' as the source of infection. Biss explains that, among the mothers with whom she talked, there was a widespread diffuse sense of mistrust. The government was inept, the mass media couldn't be trusted and business interests corrupted everything. Even the language had become corrupted. All that talk of 'herd immunity', she writes 'invites an unfortunate association with the term *herd mentality*, a stampede towards stupidity. The herd, we assume, is stupid.'[12] Who or what to believe? The world of educated middle-class professionals in which she moves is riddled with doubt, with anxiety, with contradictory information, and with mistrust of public as well as private institutions. But also with a sense of living in a protected and privileged world so that, as Biss puts it, 'The belief that public health measures are not intended for people like us is widely held by many people like me.'[13] And though she does take her son to be vaccinated, her book makes abundantly clear how her decisions are made in the face of uncertainty, of doubt. And she wants us to understand how it could hardly be otherwise, given the culture she inherits and the sense of mistrust, of betrayal even, which has become so dispiriting a feature of the world in which she lives.

Ethical reflection is supposed to help us make 'good' decisions. What kind of reflection can help us live with the decisions we have made, and with the doubts we had when making them?

How We Got to Where We Are

Investments made in vaccines and vaccinations today are vast. It is hardly surprising that the purchase of millions of doses of vaccine – selling for anything between a few cents and a hundred or more pounds, euros or dollars per shot – has created a global market now said to be worth some $25 billion per annum, and rising fast.

But there's also a vast emotional investment in a technology that we hope will protect our children from harm and possible death. And for ministers of health and their public health advisers, there is a political investment too, since mounting a national vaccination campaign can mean putting one's reputation on the line. Of course, if it can be shown afterwards that many lives have been saved, there is credit to be had. But if the outcome proves to be very different from what had been predicted and feared, someone has to be held responsible.

In February 1976 an influenza virus that appeared similar to the one that caused the 1918 Spanish flu pandemic – on which more later – was found in a military recruit at Fort Dix, New Jersey. The u.s. government's advisory committee on immunization recommended a national immunization programme against what became known as 'swine flu'. The director of the Center for Disease Control (CDC) advised that the federal government immediately contract with the pharmaceutical industry to produce sufficient vaccine to vaccinate the whole population. With a presidential election coming up, the White House became involved. After convening a high-level meeting, President Gerald Ford announced in a press conference that he had accepted these recommendations. A National Influenza Immunization Program (NIIP) was launched, and at a cost of $137 million, more than forty million Americans were immunized. Unfortunately the vaccine had side effects: 54 people were diagnosed with the neurological condition Guillain-Barré syndrome as a result of the vaccine. What is more, the suspected pandemic did not materialize. Only one person, an army recruit, died from that flu in 1976. In December of the same year the NIIP was cancelled. The incoming president, Jimmy Carter, and his secretary of health, education and welfare, Joseph Califano, decided that the director of the CDC would have to go. Credit, credibility and millions of dollars had been wasted.

What is the relevance of stories like this? Writing in 2006, Richard Krause, who had been involved in the 1976 swine flu debacle, drew a lesson for public health decision-makers confronted by similar uncertainties:

Now any number of national and international organizations and the ministries of health in many countries in Southeast

Asia are on the firing line in regard to avian influenza. Should we stockpile drugs? Prepare a vaccine? Cull infected flocks? When difficult choices arise, criticism is almost certain to follow, but as Harry Truman said, 'If you can't stand the heat, stay out of the kitchen.'[14]

When faced with the avian or later 'swine flu' epidemics, if any of his successors read this it will surely bring a wry smile to their faces. But drawing parallels that can serve as warning lessons is not the only reason for looking back. I suspect we can all recall moments that made us ask, 'How did I get *here?*' It can sometimes be helpful. For example when I'm lost I ask which street, or which path, brought me to this place. Trying to retrace my steps seems a promising way of returning to more familiar ground. Or in a conversation, surprised to find myself discussing an event or a person, I might wonder how we'd got to that. What sequence brought us here? The trigger might be simple curiosity, or it might be the wish to get back to the subject of talk before we let ourselves be diverted. Was there a distinct point at which I took a wrong turn? In walking, in talking, we can return to that point and proceed differently. In the longer term, in living one's life, it is more complicated. There may be no such point. Things build up. 'You know how it is ... one thing leads to another.' Nevertheless, asking the question can still be enlightening. Autobiography has something of the same: an exploration of the experiences through which I became what I am. Or through which I think I became what I think I am. What of public affairs? Is any purpose served by examining how we got to where we are as a community, society or polity? Or to be more specific, what could we learn from inquiring into how public health became so dependent on vaccination, or into how it came to seem responsible to protect the health of a small vulnerable child by introducing pathogenic matter into its body? What I think we will discover is that attitudes to vaccination, both positive and negative, have deep roots, and that vaccines serve more functions than we might intuitively believe to be the case.

Though modern public health relies to a considerable extent on vaccinating people, the history of public health begins long before there were any vaccines. As the governments of municipalities, states or nations began to concern themselves with protecting their populations against infection, they tended to rely on one of two approaches. Some authorities inclined to a 'contagionist' approach. Seeking to disrupt the transmission of infection they emphasized limiting the mobility of people likely to be infected, through quarantining them and their goods and chattels. 'Sanitationists', by contrast, emphasized the need to improve the conditions under which people lived and worked, so that for them the important thing was killing germs through cleaning and disinfecting. An influential view among historians of medicine has been that the former approach fitted well with, and tended to be adopted by, authoritarian systems of government, as in Prussia, while liberal-democratic political systems, such as the British, preferred the sanitationist approach.

In the second half of the nineteenth century the view gained ground that diseases are caused by specific biological entities, or 'germs'. The birth of a new science of bacteriology didn't provoke an immediate revolution in thinking about public health, though it fitted more easily with a contagionist view. But while it was becoming more difficult to claim that dirt and poverty alone could be the cause of disease, knowledge of microorganisms did not rule out a role for environmental factors or for sanitary measures. It was rather that both approaches tended to be modified in the light of the new discoveries. Sanitary measures alone would not be sufficient for controlling the spread of infection. On the other hand many of those versed in the new science doubted that traditional forms of quarantine were necessary, given that infected individuals could now be identified by the presence of germs in their bodies. Science was one thing, however, and politics was another. Historian Peter Baldwin has shown how, at the start of the twentieth century, the Great Powers often supported quarantine as a way of restricting the trade of competitor nations.[15] Nor was there agreement as to which countries could be relied upon to implement appropriate hygienic measures themselves. No less important in sustaining the use of quarantine as a tool of public health, Baldwin shows, was public opinion. Quarantine made the citizens of some countries, some cities even, feel safe, and for that reason was politically difficult to abandon. As of course is still the case, a century later.

So how did vaccines fit in? My edition of the *Oxford English Dictionary* tells me that the first written use of the term 'vaccinate' occurred in 1803, and that what it then meant was 'to inoculate with the virus of cow-pox as a protection against small-pox'.[16] The very word 'vaccine' comes from the Latin word for a cow. The story behind the origins of the term and practice has been told many times.

In the second half of the eighteenth century, smallpox – so named much earlier to differentiate it from syphilis, which produced 'great pokkes' – claimed the lives of tens of thousands of people each year in Britain alone, and as many as a million in Europe. Most victims were children. Many victims were crippled or disfigured. But through the early years of the nineteenth century, smallpox death rates were dramatically reduced. The person generally acknowledged as the hero of the story is Edward Jenner, an English country doctor. H. J. Parish, in his classic *History of Immunization*, tells a slightly more complex story.[17] According to Parish a Dorset farmer, Benjamin Jesty, was the first to try it out on his family, having noticed that two servants who had caught cowpox thereafter seemed immune to smallpox. Twenty years later, Edward Jenner, a Gloucestershire doctor, set out, more scientifically, to test what had become a widespread popular belief that catching cowpox protected against smallpox. In 1796 Jenner was able to show that if fluid was taken from one person's cowpox lesion and rubbed into the scratched-open skin of another person's arm, the second person was also protected against smallpox. It wasn't necessary to have a sick cow at hand. The matter so transferred was called 'humanized lymph', 'lymph' being a Greek word meaning a pure clear stream. As we saw, it is still the name given to the transparent fluid that carries certain cells around the body. Jenner's results were tested by leading London doctors, and by 1800 vaccination with humanized lymph had been adopted by numerous smallpox hospitals, and some 100,000 people had received it worldwide. It acquired powerful and important support from Napoleon and U.S. president Thomas Jefferson. At Jenner's urging, a National Vaccine Establishment was set up in London in 1808, under the auspices of the Royal College of Physicians. Its task was to supply lymph, as requested, throughout Britain, to its colonies and (occasionally) to other European countries. It soon had difficulty in keeping up with demand and – equally challenging – in ensuring that the lymph hadn't deteriorated by the time it reached some distant destination. Not that everyone was convinced. Many people, including many physicians and scientists, thought the idea of deliberately introducing a potentially harmful substance into people's bodies – even children's bodies – either absurd or wicked.

Advisers to the king of Spain came up with an innovative solution to the transportation problem. In 1802 the king of Spain, whose family had been affected by the disease, learned that some of Spain's colonies were facing devastating smallpox epidemics. A vaccination expedition left Spain in November 1803. On board the ship were 22 orphaned children, for the vaccine (lymph) would be passed from one child to the other in order to ensure that it remained active when the expedition reached South America a few months later. When, subsequently, the Spanish emperor instructed the expedition to continue from Mexico to the Philippines (and later to Macau and Canton), the original Spanish children (who remained in Mexico) were replaced by 25 Mexican orphans. In each place it visited, this Spanish expedition attempted to organize both systematic vaccination and local production of lymph, though with varying success. Only later would local production come to be seen as the only viable solution.

Not only was lymph made widely available, but a number of governments also made inoculation obligatory, with penalties for those who refused. Death and disfigurement from smallpox decreased, but that was not the only consequence of the smallpox vaccination programmes that were set up around the world.

Jenner's discovery, and the work of the pioneering bacteriologists, which we will discuss in the next chapter, laid the foundations for modern vaccinology: the development and production of more and better vaccines. Looking back, it is relatively easy to construct a narrative of progress – scientific, technological and medical – from all that has happened since. This is how the history of science and technology is generally presented, so it seems familiar. But it is not the only narrative that can be drawn from the history of vaccines and vaccination. If we look more critically we soon recognize other themes, other potential narratives. One might concern the uses of vaccines. How have vaccines been used, taken to the people (usually children) whom they are to protect? How was vaccination related to other medical actions or services? Who decided which vaccines were to be given, and to whom, and on what basis did they decide?

Was vaccination to be voluntary or was there to be an element of compulsion? What of popular sentiments and perceptions? For most parents, in the industrialized world at least, it has become normal, the default option, to take children to be vaccinated. How did this come about, given that vaccines are (or were) made from nasty biological materials? How 'stable' are the views that lie behind this 'normal behaviour'? Are there not times when fear destabilizes it, leading to enhanced demand (even, in its filmic versions, obsessive demand)? And how universal is it? In most societies people have access to what we might call a 'repertoire of cultural resources' for thinking about vaccines and vaccinations. These repertoires, not everywhere the same, depend on past interventions and experiences that have impressed themselves on the collective memory. Feeling threatened and panicky, we inhabitants of modern industrial societies might view vaccination as our only hope. Indifference, passive acceptance, is an alternative way of thinking about it, and by far the most common. But in most countries there are some people who refuse vaccination, implying that doubt and rejection represent another sentiment available to us. Details change, and the ways in which enthusiasm or doubts are formulated change; but all have deep roots.

All that later became known about the bacterial causes of disease notwithstanding, when an epidemic breaks out there seems to be a deeply rooted need to blame some distinctive 'others'. As Roy Porter pointed out at the start of the AIDS epidemic, 'When the tabloids scream about the gay plague', there was no doubt about who was to be held responsible for people's fear: a message forcefully exploited by the tabloid press.[18] Stigmatization is unwelcome, and just as the gay community reacted to being blamed for – as well as suffering exceedingly from – the AIDS epidemic, so did 'the great unwashed' protest a century earlier. However scared of becoming infected with smallpox people may have been in the nineteenth century, they did not all welcome the start of the compulsory vaccination campaigns that were being established. Resistance emerged. In 1871 the government of the Netherlands reacted to an epidemic of smallpox by requiring that all schoolchildren be vaccinated. Widespread resistance crystallized a few years later in the formation of a League to Oppose Compulsory Vaccination. The opposition wasn't so much to vaccination per se as to the compulsion. With many clerics among its members the league considered compulsory vaccination an infringement of individual liberty. (By the early years of the twentieth century the view that religious beliefs constituted a valid reason for refusing vaccination had become accepted in the Netherlands, and remains so to this day.) In the United States resistance also became particularly strong in the 1870s and '80s, though the motives of those who established anti-vaccination societies there appear to have been slightly different from those of the Dutch. Many leaders of these associations in the United States were 'irregular physicians' (including homeopaths), who felt their ability to practise would be threatened by state intervention.

Opposition arose in England and Wales too, as laws passed between 1853 and 1871 made vaccination of infants against smallpox compulsory. Those who could afford the services of a medical practitioner were far less inconvenienced by these laws than were poor people. Parents who could not afford to go to a GP were directed to state-paid vaccinators who functioned under the aegis of the Poor Law Guardians. This in itself was cruelly stigmatizing, since the whole Poor Law administration was deeply hated. Even worse, Poor Law vaccinators had the task of seeking out and prosecuting poor parents who failed to comply with the law. As historian Nadja Durbach has shown, there was a deep resentment among working-class people about the increasing 'disciplining of the body' by the state, of which this appeared to be one facet.[19] Middle-class liberal anti-vaccinationists principally objected to the erosion of individual liberty entailed in compulsory vaccination. The thousands of respectable working-class anti-vaccinationists had different objections. They found each other, however, in an anti-vaccination movement that emerged in the 1860s. Durbach shows how both proponents of vaccination, and its opponents, appealed to notions of good citizenship. Vaccinating for the one was an obligation that went with being a good citizen. It was to protect the community from disease. For the other, however, citizenship entailed respecting the body of one's neighbour, rather than (as one activist quoted by Durbach pointed out) 'legalizing bodily assault'. For many of the working-class members of the Anti-compulsory Vaccination League and other similar organizations, rejection of vaccination was of a piece with the other 'lifestyle choices' they made: abstinence from alcohol, vegetarianism, membership of self-help organizations and trades unionism.

In England too much of the resistance to vaccination focused on the element of compulsion, rather than on vaccination itself. Protestors claimed the right to opt out for reasons of conscience. In many places these societies were able to bring about the repeal of compulsory vaccination laws. Thereafter they started to decline. For example, in Britain the government responded to public discontent by appointing a Royal Commission on Vaccination in 1889. It sat for seven years before coming up with compromise proposals, though it took until 1907 before the law was changed to allow for a right to opt out.

A focus on policies, or on public opinion, provides an alternative way of writing the story of how vaccines came to occupy the place they do in public health, in politics, in the economy and in culture. There is a simple reason why the 'scientific' story, the story of progress, is so much more familiar than these. A history that shows increasingly sophisticated tools being crafted to vanquish one terrible disease after another is a story that offers comfort and holds out hope. It reflects an idea of public health grounded in science, rather than in politics or in economics, which offer neither comfort nor hope. It is also a useful history, regularly deployed to justify faith in the future promise of vaccines and in the need to invest in them today.

What is the point of trying to subvert these accounts with others? Why try to write alternative histories of vaccines and vaccination? Perhaps it is easier to see with some different examples. Think of computers. Of course we could write a history of miniaturization, of the computing power that ever-smaller devices can be made to yield, looking forward to biocomputing and the post-silicon economy. But who would find that a technical history like that offers much insight into what from a social or cultural perspective is most important about computers and information technology: the way they have influenced personal, social and working life?

Or to stay in the same general area . . . think about the social media that have become so ubiquitous. What do they do? Well, they enable social networking and that's why people join: to keep up with all their 'friends' and feed their 'followers' – to the extent that not joining may have to be explained and justified on all sides, while leaving, an act of abandonment or betrayal, is likely to be greeted with horror. Is that all that is to be said? Clearly not. There is a business story – stock market flotations and profits. And as we now know, there is a security story. Who is collecting and collating the personal data that millions of people so liberally strew around, and for what purposes? Many stories can be told of a technology, and there may be powerful interests in promoting one perspective and one such story, at the expense of other perspectives and the alternative stories to which they lead. A major objective of some of the most important social movements of the twentieth century was to articulate and promote alternative stories about being female, gay or disabled, or about nuclear power, or destruction of the natural environment. Things, practices, that have been 'naturalized' over time, made to seem self-evident, inevitable or invisible, had to be stripped of their cultural accretions and looked at differently. Artists have recognized this for two hundred years. Sociologists, when they discovered it, referred to it as 'reframing'.

Almost all technologies can be used in all sorts of ways, and how effective they are will depend on what they are used for. Think of a screwdriver being used to prise open a door or unblock a plughole! Vaccines are no different. Maybe that sounds odd. Surely limiting the spread of an infectious disease is the only purpose of a vaccine?

Absolutely not. Perhaps that was the case when smallpox vaccination began – though from the perspective of those who protested against compulsory vaccination it was an attempt to discipline the working class or restrict individual freedoms. In the course of time, 'vaccination' lost its specific association with smallpox, so that a century later a vaccine was 'a preparation of some virus used for the purposes of inoculation'. Laws changed, smallpox declined (in Europe at least) and organized resistance diminished. At the same time, underlying sentiments, associations and significances also changed. My dictionary also tells me that in 1892 the author and political activist Israel Zangwill wrote in his novel *Children of the Ghetto*, 'Who will vaccinate him against free-thinking, as I would have done?'[20] Clearly Zangwill wasn't thinking of cowpox here. He was writing at a time at which scientists in Berlin and Paris were developing a new science of bacteriology, and the prospect of effectively combatting infectious diseases was in the air. When Zangwill wrote about 'vaccination against free-thinking', he was speaking metaphorically. By the time he wrote, the idea of vaccination was no longer linked uniquely to the prevention of smallpox. Vaccinations against other diseases (anthrax, rabies) were known and had been used. But vaccinating against something going on in an individual's mind?

Between May 2013 and May 2014 more than seven hundred clinical trials of vaccines were in progress, being conducted in more than sixty countries (though directed by scientists from just a handful of countries). Some of these trials have nothing whatever to do with limiting the spread of infectious diseases. In a few trials candidate vaccines are being tested that should render someone infertile, or immune to an addiction to nicotine or cocaine. As vaccines are gradually being transformed into *technologies of risk avoidance*, Zangwill's metaphor is slowly becoming reality.

TWO

TECHNOLOGIES: THE FIRST VACCINES

With his famous description of the living conditions of the nineteenth-century urban poor, Friedrich Engels evoked the conditions under which hundreds of thousands of people struggled to survive. Here is part of his description of what he found in Manchester:

> Everywhere half or wholly ruined buildings, some of them actually uninhabited, which means a great deal here; rarely a wooden or stone floor to be seen in the houses, almost uniformly broken, ill-fitting windows and doors, and a state of filth! Everywhere heaps of debris, refuse, and offal; standing pools for gutters, and a stench which alone would make it impossible for a human being in any degree civilised to live in such a district. The newly-built extension of the Leeds railway, which crosses the Irk here, has swept away some of these courts and lanes, laying others completely open to view. Immediately under the railway bridge there stands a court, the filth and horrors of which surpass all the others by far, just because it was hitherto so shut off, so secluded that the way to it could not be found without a good deal of trouble. I should never have discovered it myself, without the breaks made by the railway, though I thought I knew this whole region thoroughly. Passing along a rough bank, among stakes and washing-lines, one penetrates into this chaos of small one-storied, one-roomed huts, in most of which there is no artificial floor; kitchen, living and sleeping-room all in one. In such a hole, scarcely five feet long by six broad, I found two

beds – and such bedsteads and beds! – which, with a staircase and chimney-place, exactly filled the room. In several others I found absolutely nothing, while the door stood open, and the inhabitants leaned against it. Everywhere before the doors refuse and offal; that any sort of pavement lay underneath could not be seen but only felt, here and there, with the feet. This whole collection of cattle-sheds for human beings was surrounded on two sides by houses and a factory, and on the third by the river, and besides the narrow stair up the bank, a narrow doorway alone led out into another almost equally ill-built, ill-kept labyrinth of dwellings.[1]

Engels's description of living conditions in 1844 was still applicable for decades thereafter. A child born in Manchester in the 1870s could expect to live only for 34 years, its London-born contemporary for a mere six years more. Drawing on hospital records, death certificates and other contemporary material, historians have spent a great deal of time and energy trying to disentangle the causes of nineteenth-century sickness and mortality. One of the things that has made their task difficult is that the ways in which diseases are characterized and distinguished one from the other have changed over time. Because they could show similar symptoms – fevers, diarrhoea – diseases that later came to be seen as distinct were long confused one with the other. Moreover, the patterns historians have uncovered are not uniform. It is difficult to generalize. In some places, at some times, poor areas of cities suffered far more disease than rich areas. At other times and in other places this was not so. In some places at some times the illness experience of city dwellers was far worse than that of their country cousins. At other times, in other places, the difference was small. What is clear, however, is that a great deal of sickness and death in large cities – perhaps as much as 50 per cent – was due to infectious disease. The squalid, insanitary and overcrowded conditions in which the majority of the urban poor were forced to live meant that infectious respiratory and gastro-enteric diseases spread easily and rapidly. This was especially true among soldiers at war, crowded together in filthy camps. In late nineteenth-century wars (such as the Crimean War and the Franco–Prussian War), more soldiers died of infectious disease than in combat. Engels was not alone in his horrified response to the filth and overcrowding he found in British cities. Edwin Chadwick's famous *Report on the Sanitary Condition of the Labouring Population of Great Britain*, which appeared in 1842, brought public health firmly onto the political agenda.[2] Industrialization, in full swing in late nineteenth-century Britain, also played its part. Because it is so disruptive, and in so many ways, the start of industrialization has always brought threats to health with it, and these threats weigh most heavily on the impoverished and the marginalized.

Because many of the diseases that afflicted ill-fed and impoverished populations shared similar symptoms, they were difficult to identify with any certainty. Symptoms of feverish headaches, followed by a rash spreading over most of the body, and then by sensitivity to light, and delirium and probably death, were likely to be typhus. Typhus was later found to be carried by lice, and despite the similar names, to be quite distinct from another scourge of the time, typhoid. Typhus is said to have been particularly common in nineteenth-century Glasgow, referred to by historian Michael Flinn as being 'possibly the filthiest and unhealthiest of all the British towns' in the mid-nineteenth century.[3] In the 1830s, Europe was therefore all the more shaken by another disease, which seemed to strike preferentially at more affluent neighbourhoods and not the most impoverished ones. Its symptoms, notably watery diarrhoea, which could lead to dehydration and death, meant that for many years it could not be distinguished from other infections of the bowel. When cholera – for that is what it was – first arrived in Western Europe it evoked terror and despair. No one knew what it was or where it had come from. By the time it returned, in 1865, more was known of the origins and movement of the disease. Investigators had discovered that epidemics typically originated near to the great rivers of India and China. Carried westward by returning pilgrims, immigrant labourers and trading vessels, it easily fed into the dread, and the racialized horror, captured at the end of the nineteenth century by the term the 'yellow peril'. Improved means of transportation (steamships across the Mediterranean, railways and later the Suez Canal) only added to the threat. Soon after the 1865 epidemic in Europe, a ship travelling from Marseilles to New York introduced the disease to the Americas.

The greatest killer of all was tuberculosis, also known as consumption, as phthisis, and as hectic fever. Though tuberculosis (TB) was everywhere, thriving in the debilitated bodies of the ill-nourished and the overworked, its sentimentalized image obscured its association with poverty and malnutrition. In the nineteenth-century artistic and popular imagination, tuberculosis was widely associated with Romantics and Romanticism. The poet John Keats died of it aged only 26, his lungs at autopsy found to be almost completely destroyed. Chopin suffered from TB, as did Shelley, Paganini, Robert Louis Stevenson, Henry David Thoreau, Emerson and all of the Brontës. Because it seemed to run in certain families there was a widespread view that it was due to an inherited sensitivity, or susceptibility. Some saw it as somehow associated with aesthetic creativity. In their classic study of tuberculosis, René and Jean Dubos quote Thoreau (writing in 1852): 'Decay and disease are often beautiful, like . . . the hectic glow of consumption.'[4] The ideal of feminine beauty – languid, pallid – which inspired Edgar Allen Poe and the Pre-Raphaelite painters, and which Dubos refers to as an 'attitude of perverted sentimentalism toward tuberculosis', gave way only towards the end of the nineteenth century:

> Turning their eyes away from the languorous fainting young women and their romantic lovers [poets and writers] noticed instead the miserable humanity living in the dreary tenements of the Industrial Revolution . . . Tuberculosis was there, breeding suffering and misery without romance.[5]

The poets, painters and writers who died of tuberculosis were hardly representative victims of a disease that probably accounted for a third of all deaths in England and Wales (and doubtless elsewhere) in the first half of the nineteenth century.

There was a single exception to this bleak picture. By the mid-nineteenth century it was becoming clear that inoculation with Jenner's vaccine had greatly reduced death and serious illness resulting from smallpox. Jenner had even claimed that the technique would lead to eradication of the disease – as indeed it did, though two hundred years later! So why not tackle other infectious diseases – tuberculosis, typhus, typhoid, cholera and (especially threatening in the Americas) yellow fever in the same way?

The possibility of combatting smallpox with Jenner's vaccine had depended on a chance observation, subsequently confirmed, that exposure to a mild animal disease (cowpox) could protect humans against a related but much more serious disease (smallpox). Would the same approach work with the other infectious diseases that threatened human life in the nineteenth century? Would it only be possible if a closely related but milder animal disease could be found? It was the great French chemist Louis Pasteur who showed that the answer to this question is 'no': that there are other ways of producing this protective effect. Turning from his early work on crystallography, Pasteur began to study fermentation and other processes, which he showed were due to the growth of microorganisms. The heat treatment of milk or other beverages in order to kill microorganisms that would spoil them became known as 'pasteurization' in honour of Pasteur's achievement in this field.

Pasteur realized that cultures of microorganisms could be attenuated, or weakened, and that infection with this weakened microorganism should protect against later challenge by the virulent form. What he did not understand at first was how this attenuation could best be brought about, and he investigated a number of procedures, working first on anthrax, primarily a disease of animals. He prepared cultures of the bacillus, attenuated them by exposure to air or by treatment with chemicals, and tried these out on rabbits and sheep, and later on cattle and horses. His public demonstration in May 1881, at Pouilly-le-Fort, attracted widespread publicity. Much still had to be learned regarding the stability of the weakened bacillus, and how it could be produced to a standard potency. Nevertheless, Pasteur's laboratory soon embarked on large-scale production, and within a year thousands of sheep had been inoculated, with considerable effect on anthrax mortality. Pasteur called the immunity-producing culture a 'vaccine' as a tribute to Jenner. Through the 1880s hundreds of thousands of doses were produced each year in the central production facility that Pasteur established in Paris. Together with his colleagues Emile Roux and Charles Chamberland, Pasteur then went on to study rabies, which in humans is generally caused by the bite of an infected animal. The organism responsible was so small that they were unable to see it under the microscope, and nor could they grow it in glass dishes (*in vitro*). However, they were able to establish that it multiplied in the spinal cord and brain of infected animals. Having injected matter taken from an infected animal into the brain of another animal, they discovered that many such 'passages' through monkey brains decreased the virulence for dogs and rabbits. This was a different way of 'attenuating' from the one they had used for their anthrax vaccine, but it now seemed that a vaccine against rabies was also within reach. The next step was to see how it could best be produced on a larger scale.

By 1884 they had settled on a procedure that involved infecting rabbits, waiting until they died, removing their spinal cords, drying these in sterile air for two weeks and then grinding them to a powder. Vaccine was prepared by emulsifying small portions of powdered spinal cord in salt solution. In this way dogs could be protected. Pasteur and his colleagues didn't yet understand how precisely the attenuation worked, but from a public health perspective this was less important than the fact that it did, in practice, work. There was a good deal of resistance in the medical profession to the idea of trying out this concoction on humans, and Emile Roux, who unlike Pasteur was a medical doctor, was reluctant to take that step. Despite Roux's doubts, in 1885 a boy named Joseph Meister, who had received what was thought to be a fatal bite from a rabid dog, was treated with it. According to Parish, Meister soon recovered and later became the porter at the Pasteur Institute. Not everyone was so fortunate. It later turned out that success or failure depended on how soon after having been bitten a patient was treated. Rabies has a long incubation period, and to be saved the patient had to be treated before infection reached the central nervous system. Thereafter other researchers tried to produce a better rabies vaccine, by varying the drying process, or by chemically treating the substance they extracted from the brains of rabbits. This phenolized, or 'killed', vaccine could be kept for several months without losing its protective qualities.

Jenner and Pasteur had established the principle of vaccination, and Pasteur had shown that by weakening, or attenuating, a bacillus, a protective serum could be made. In Pasteur's laboratory in Paris, and in that directed by Robert Koch in Berlin, a new science of bacteriology was taking shape. Not that the institutions they directed shared an identical vision either of how the field should develop or of the theoretical basis of their endeavours. Pasteur's ideas regarding the mechanism of disease causation, and in particular the influence of environmental factors, differed substantially from those of Koch.

So too did the structure of the institutes that they directed, reflecting the different political and administrative traditions of the two countries (which had actually been at war with one another only a decade earlier). The institute established in honour of Pasteur (Institut Pasteur, founded in 1888) and that established for Koch (Institut für Infektionskrankheiten, or Institute for Infectious Diseases, founded in 1891) had very different structures and were organized and financed very differently. The Paris institute had an endowment fund, much of which came from the donations of the French public. The Berlin institute was established and funded by the state, and organized as hierarchically as any other Prussian institution. These structural differences, as well more general differences in policies and attitudes regarding science and industry, would soon affect both how they related to each other and how and where the new vaccines were manufactured in each of the two countries.

It was from these two centres, from Paris and Berlin, that investigations of the bacterial causes of diseases spread outwards. Physicians came to Paris or Berlin from far and wide to follow the training courses given there, or they read about the new science and began to experiment by themselves. After the rabies announcement, doctors came from nearby countries and returned home with rabbits inoculated according to Pasteur's instruction. From more distant countries came representatives of the state: the emperor of Brazil, the Ottoman Sultan, the czar of Russia. There were also local physicians far from Berlin or Paris, who were intrigued by what they had read of the new bacteriology. One was a Cuban physician, Carlos Finlay, who in the 1880s was the first to suggest that yellow fever is carried by a mosquito. Pasteur's work on anthrax and rabies had shown that vaccines against diseases other than smallpox were effective, but these were not major sources of human disease and death. If bacteriology was to be put to use in controlling the many infectious scourges of nineteenth-century life, then the causative agent of each separate disease would first have to be identified.

Practitioners of the new bacteriology looked for the bacterial causes responsible for so much of the disease they saw all around them. In 1880 a bacillus named *Salmonella typhi* was identified as the cause of typhoid. In 1882 Robert Koch found the bacillus responsible for tuberculosis, and a few years later Albert Klebs in Zurich identified and isolated the one that caused diphtheria. But identifying, isolating and successfully culturing the bacillus is only the start. In order to produce a protective vaccine they would have to go on to isolate and sufficiently attenuate a strain of the bacillus. Getting the attenuation right was crucial, since if the bacillus hadn't been weakened sufficiently the culture could still be poisonous. If the process went on for too long it might well lose its protective qualities. When researchers thought they had got it right, the proto-vaccine would then have to be tested on humans (who might or might not be volunteers). And if all of that worked, and if it could be shown to work, it would have to be made on a large scale. Large-scale production raised different issues, of ensuring standard and consistent potency and quality.

This was, roughly speaking, the pattern. Researchers, almost all working in public or semi-public institutions, tried to isolate the pathogens responsible for some of the major threats to public health of their time, and then to find the best way of attenuating them. If the proto-vaccine appeared effective, production would somehow have to be scaled up. It took years for this to be accomplished and in most cases much longer before any of the new vaccines were actually used on a large scale. There were social as well as technical obstacles to overcome. For one thing, there was the scepticism of many who had not been convinced by the bacterial theory of disease. Especially in the case of tuberculosis there were influential physicians wholly committed to other approaches, such as the fresh-air regime practised in mountain-top sanatoria. When scepticism had eventually declined and preventive vaccination was more generally accepted, other challenges followed. If vaccines were to be used on a large scale then standards for quality and potency would have to be established. Moreover, developments in statistical methods led to more rigorous tests of effectiveness.

Applying Bacteriology: Crafting Vaccines

Diphtheria is an infection of the upper respiratory tract, with symptoms that include sore throat, coughing and difficulties in breathing and swallowing. A characteristic of the disease is the formation of a membrane that covers the tonsils and pharynx. In the nineteenth century it was a devastating disease of children, though adults were rarely affected. Common treatments at the time included regular scrubbing of the throat, inhaling various vapours that were thought to be beneficial and, in the most serious cases, tracheotomy (the opening of the windpipe to enable the victim to breathe without using their nose or mouth). Klebs's identification of the bacteria causing diphtheria, subsequently confirmed by Friedrich Loeffler, an assistant to Koch, had major implications. It would now be possible to diagnose the disease by bacteriological analysis rather than by relying on symptoms that overlapped with those of other diseases. Having discovered that the bacillus kills by producing a poison, known as a toxin, Loeffler's proposal was for 'internal disinfection' (gargling). However, it was Emil Behring and the Japanese bacteriologist Shibasaburo Kitasato, working in Koch's laboratory, who in 1890 discovered an antidote. They found that when small amounts of the poison produced in culturing the bacilli were injected into healthy animals, the animals produced a neutralizing serum that could then be used to kill diphtheria bacilli. The serum became known as an 'antitoxin'. The animals that had received it became immune. This was shown by challenging them with lethal doses. At the end of 1891 a little girl was successfully treated with antitoxin prepared in a sheep.

By this time both the Berlin and Paris groups had independently established that serum taken from immunized animals neutralized the diphtheria toxin, though they had different theories as to how this worked or what it implied. Was this protective effect the same as 'immunity' (as Behring argued), or was immunity a different process to be understood in terms of what Roux and his colleague Metschnikoff called 'phagocytosis', from the Greek word *phagein*, to devour? For the French, the serum worked not by neutralizing the toxin but by stimulating cells to 'engulf' an invading particle (a so-called phagocytic reaction).

Different investigators worked with different animals. While Behring used sheep to produce serum, other German researchers, working along parallel lines, used dogs. The larger the animal the more blood serum it would produce, and it was Roux and his colleagues in Paris who showed how serum could be produced on a much larger scale using horses rather than sheep or dogs. Diphtheria bacilli, grown on a special medium, were killed and used to immunize the animals. It was tricky because the process, and hence the strength of the toxin, varied with all sorts of factors, including the strain of bacterium, the culture medium and the temperature at which the culture was maintained. After ten or so inoculations, spread over weeks or months, and when the horse was thought to have produced enough antitoxin, five or six litres of blood were collected from each horse. The blood was then filtered and centrifuged to separate the serum.

With their serum, Roux and colleagues were able to halve the number of deaths from diphtheria in the Paris Hôpital des Enfants Malades. This achievement rapidly became known abroad, exciting considerable interest. The Pasteur Institute established a facility to produce serum on a larger scale. In 1894 Roux's serum was used for the first time in England. Sir Joseph Lister had obtained some during a visit to Paris and given it to a London hospital, where it was used successfully to treat twenty patients. In the same year, Armand Ruffer, an ex-pupil of Pasteur, prepared some at the British Institute of Preventive Medicine, recently established in London with the support of the Guinness family (it was later renamed the Jenner Institute and subsequently the Lister Institute). Elsewhere in London, Ruffer and Sir Charles Sherrington were producing serum in a horse (the BIPM had no space for so large an animal), and in October 1894 Sherrington administered it to an eight-year-old boy who was thought to be dying from diphtheria. He recovered. In hospitals where diphtheria patients were treated with antitoxin the death rate fell dramatically in the years leading up to the First World War. Though this serum treatment was referred to as 'vaccination' because of the way it was administered, what was involved wasn't preventive immunization as we think of it today. Preventive vaccination against diphtheria would only become a serious possibility some years later, as a result of further developments.

A dose of antitoxin did confer some protection against the disease, but only for a very short time. This is when researchers gradually came to understand the difference between what became known as 'passive' and 'active' immunity. Antibodies introduced into the body from outside provide only short-lived immunity. But if the body could be stimulated to produce the antibodies itself, the resulting active immunity would persist for very much longer. The next step was development of a method of active immunization. Parish credits Behring (who changed his name to 'von Behring' after winning the Nobel Prize in 1901) with this through his continued use of toxin–antitoxin mixture and his demonstration (in 1913) that in this way lasting immunity could be produced in humans. The second development was the achievement of Bela Schick, a Hungarian paediatrician working at the University of Vienna. Schick developed a test, used in Britain for the first time in 1922, for determining whether an individual is susceptible to diphtheria. A very small dose of toxin is injected into the skin. A reddening of the skin at the injection site shows the patient is susceptible; lack of reaction that they are immune. Since it was believed the serum could be harmful to people who were already immune, the Schick test saved many people being given the injection. The third important development involved replacement of the toxin–antitoxin mixtures, which were still being used, but which could be dangerous. In 1924 Gaston Ramon at the Pasteur Institute discovered that when diphtheria toxin was treated with formalin it produced a substance, a 'toxoid', that was no longer virulent but which still stimulated antitoxin production. Ramon called it 'anatoxine' and urged that this be used in place of the toxin–antitoxin mixtures. After trials had been done and it had been approved by the Academy of Medicine, its use spread. With the replacement of toxin by toxoid, vaccination became much safer.

However, while toxoid was rapidly absorbed at the site of injection, it was also rapidly eliminated. This led to studies of how it could be kept longer in the body, and the discovery of what became known as 'adjuvants'. Building on further work by Ramon, in 1926 researchers at the Wellcome laboratories in London found that if alum (a simple chemical compound, potassium aluminium sulphate) were added to the toxoid it remained in tissue for much longer. It was this purified 'alum-precipitated toxoid' that eventually entered widespread use. It is important to understand how much research was needed, how many challenges had to be faced, before prophylactic vaccination came to be seen as a feasible and efficacious manner of protecting large numbers of children against diphtheria. The move from therapeutic use of the toxin–antitoxin to prophylactic use depended upon a growing understanding of immunity, as well as on a number of empirical developments (the safer toxoid, development of the first adjuvant). These new perceptions were profoundly to influence the process of vaccine development. But, as the many years it took to develop a vaccine against tuberculosis show all too well, that did not mean that it would suddenly become easy or rapid.

Among the many diseases to which the early bacteriologists turned their attention, few equalled tuberculosis in the suffering it caused or the cultural resonances it evoked. Best known as a lung disease, doctors now know that it can spread to many other organs (including skin – lupus, and lymph glands in the neck – scrofula). Before the late nineteenth century, it was not known that these were all forms of a single disease. Tuberculosis was the greatest single cause of disease and death in the Western world. Though in its early (pre-symptomatic) stages, tuberculosis could not be recognized at the time, it seems likely that all inhabitants of large cities became infected at an early age. Because before the advent of bacteriological testing (and later chest X-ray) only the severest cases were found, it was impossible to tell how many people had milder infections. Though it was the single largest cause of death, tuberculosis was not commonly viewed as a 'public health' disease. Not only did 'consumption' not appear to be epidemic, but many thought that it ran in families. Heredity gave the predisposition, but actual development of the disease was triggered by cold wind, bad air or injury to bronchi or lungs.

When the idea that it was contagious, and in this respect similar to typhoid, was put forward by William Budd in the late 1860s, his suggestion found little support. Jean-Antoine Villemin, a surgeon in the French army, reached similar conclusions at about the same time and was similarly ignored. As Dubos explains, Villemin believed he had shown that 'tuberculosis does not originate spontaneously in man or animals as a result of emaciation [or] bad heredity' but rather that it was caused by 'some germ, living and multiplying in the body of the patient, and transmissible to a well person by direct contact or through the air'.[6] But because doctors were convinced that only people with a consumptive constitution, an 'innate suscep-tibility', became sick, evidence that tuberculosis was an infectious disease was ignored. Views changed, though only gradually, and by 1880 there was a growing sense that, indeed, some microorganism was responsible.

Then, in 1882, Robert Koch announced that he had found it: the tubercle bacillus. His lecture to the Physiological Society of Berlin brought him world fame. Apart from describing the cause of tuberculosis, the lecture showed *how* he had proven that this specific microorganism caused the disease. Koch showed, first, that the bacilli were present in all tuberculous lesions of both humans and animals. Second, he showed how the bacillus could be cultured in the laboratory. These principles were later to become enshrined in the so-called Koch's Postulates: the basis on which a given microorganism could be shown to be responsible for a given disease. But their initial importance was essentially practical. Tuberculosis was so important and so familiar a cause of death – far more so than the mostly rather obscure diseases that had been linked to specific bacteria prior to 1882 – that considerable expectations were now directed to the new science of bacteriology. The bacilli could be grown, albeit very slowly, in sheep or ox serum carefully sterilized and coagulated by heating to 65 degrees centigrade. Thereafter efforts to develop a tuberculosis vaccine proliferated, employing a whole variety of attenuation processes and bacilli taken from every imaginable species of animal.

In 1890, and to great fanfare, Koch went a step further. He announced that he'd developed a cure for tuberculosis, which he called tuberculin. While he refused to disclose its composition, and there was little evidence that it worked, Koch's reputation was by this time enough to guarantee it would be used. Soon articles on experience with its use began to appear: first positive, and then less so, and gradually followed by reports of deaths. Anxieties grew when, after carrying out autopsies on corpses, the renowned pathologist Rudolf Virchow showed that tuberculin did not kill the bacteria at all. Koch was eventually forced to reveal the composition of his secret cure, which turned out to be no more than an extract of tuberculosis bacilli in glycerine. Arthur Conan Doyle (a medical practitioner as well as the creator of Sherlock Holmes) was one of Koch's many eminent visitors. His assessment of 'tuberculin' was that it wouldn't cure anyone, and could even be dangerous, but that it would provide a useful diagnostic test. This proved indeed to be the case. Injected under the skin, it produced a local reaction (swelling and reddening) in people who were already infected with the tuberculosis bacterium. The tuberculin test would later become a standard means of testing for present or past tuberculosis infection, but this was not Koch's work and his reputation was damaged by the failure of his much-heralded treatment.

Meanwhile most attempts at developing a vaccine against tuberculosis were leading nowhere. The only one of the many candidate vaccines that eventually began to be used widely was developed by the Pasteur Institute. It took many years. Albert Calmette became a member of Pasteur's staff in 1890, working for a time in Vietnam. In 1895, returning to France to take up an appointment as head of a research institute in Lille, he started studying tuberculosis. Ten years later Calmette was collaborating with Camille Guérin, studying a strain of the tuberculosis bacillus taken from cows. Though some investigators at the time thought that a safe vaccine could best be made by chemically 'killing' the bacillus, Calmette and Guérin were looking at ways of attenuating it, in line with the Pasteurian tradition. Needless to say, the First World War and the German occupation of Lille caused considerable difficulties. Cattle were requisitioned by the German army and Calmette had problems with the occupying forces. Only in 1918, when the war ended, could the research move ahead again. It took thirteen years, and hundreds of subcultures, before Calmette and Guérin had obtained what seemed to be a sufficiently attenuated and stable preparation that was still antigenic enough to protect cattle against infection. By 1921 their vaccine, which had meanwhile come to be known as BCG (an abbreviation of 'Bacillus Calmette-Guérin'), was felt to be ready for a human trial. In July of that year Benjamin Weill-Hallé, a physician at the Paris Hôpital de la Charité, administered the vaccine orally to a newborn baby whose mother had died of tuberculosis. The baby remained healthy. Because there were no ill effects, a few other physicians were invited to try out the vaccine, and more babies were vaccinated with a somewhat larger dose. The effects of these vaccinations were monitored through carefully recording clinical parameters such as changes in weight and body temperature, as well as through clinical observation. Calmette did not bother with the tuberculin test since it seemed to produce mixed results. Between 1921 and 1924 the vaccine was sent to French medical practitioners around the country, without charge and in exchange for data on its effect: a 'non-monetary exchange'. In 1927 Calmette published a book in which he put all the relevant knowledge into the public domain. By this time the Pasteur Institute had also begun supplying BCG vaccine at no cost to physicians abroad. Calmette required only that countries should establish procedures for its production and distribution, and for monitoring the results. Robert Koch had discovered the tubercule bacillus in 1882, but it had taken another forty years for a vaccine based on his discovery to achieve any measure of acceptance.

In 1883 Koch travelled to Alexandria and then on to Calcutta. Applying the same method he had used with tuberculosis, he was able to isolate an organism from the intestines of cholera victims and to show that it was responsible for the disease. The organism became known as the *Vibrio cholerae* or 'comma bacillus', because of its shape when viewed under a microscope. Attempts to develop a vaccine against this frightening disease soon followed. A Spanish doctor, Jaime Ferran, may have been the first to try to vaccinate against cholera. Ferran had read of Pasteur's work, and in 1884 had travelled to investigate a cholera outbreak in southern France. On his return, Ferran succeeded in culturing the bacillus, attenuating it, and then using it when an epidemic broke out in Valencia. Many foreign scientists, including an influential French commission, dismissed Ferran's work as without merit. It didn't help his case that, hoping to exploit his discovery commercially, Ferran refused to give details of his attenuation procedure. At the same time Waldemar Haffkine was working independently along similar lines. Haffkine was a Russian Jewish political radical, who had been imprisoned for his opposition to the czarist regime. Trained in zoology, he emigrated, first to Switzerland and then to Paris. In 1890, having been invited to work as an assistant in Emile Roux's laboratory, he experimented with highly virulent cholera strains including one sent by Calmette from Vietnam, inoculating them into guinea pigs. Many leading scientists were sceptical of this work too, either because they were not convinced that *V. cholerae* was the cause of the disease, or because they doubted that anything could be learned from studying guinea pigs. But Haffkine persisted and in 1892, having tested his vaccines on himself and three friends, he announced his discovery. Haffkine was convinced that after one shot of weakened vaccine, followed a few days later by one shot of a stronger preparation, people would have become immune to cholera. Though both have a valid claim to having produced the first cholera vaccine, neither Ferran's nor Haffkine's vaccine survived. Both vaccines were later found to provoke too strong a reaction for general use.

Here was another problem that would have to be faced. This problem of 'reactogenicity' was not entirely new, having been encountered earlier by typhoid researchers. Both Richard Pfeiffer and Wilhelm Kolle in Berlin, and Almroth Wright at the British Army Medical Service, had been trying to develop a typhoid vaccine since the 1880s. Believing that a killed vaccine would be safer than an attenuated one, Wright's method involved heat-treating a broth containing the bacillus and adding a disinfectant, Lysol. His hope of trying out his vaccine had been thwarted, however, because the soldiers for whom it was intended were reluctant to volunteer. They were alarmed by the severe reactions the vaccine produced, and anti-typhoid vaccination was somewhat discredited in Britain. However, things changed again in the years leading up to the First World War. Wright's successor at the Army Medical Service, William Leishman, showed that the temperature at which the bacilli were killed was crucial. Having refined the production process, and by carefully regulating the dosage, Leishman was able to produce an effective and less 'reactogenic' vaccine.

Other diseases proved far more intractable. The first yellow fever epidemics in South America, the southern United States and the Caribbean had been described in the mid-seventeenth century. The disease had probably been taken there from Africa, via the West Indies: an unwelcome by-product of the slave trade. Striking unexpectedly at irregular intervals, with frightening symptoms and a high case fatality rate, the disease was an obvious focus of attention for bacteriologists in the Americas and the Caribbean. They made little progress, however, because all attempts at isolating the pathogen failed. It would be decades before a yellow fever vaccine was within reach.

Organizing Vaccine Production at the Turn of the Century

Producing a serum or a vaccine in useful quantities, let alone demonstrating that it both worked and was safe, posed all kinds of problems. An individual researcher could engage in bacteriological investigation with the aid of a simple laboratory, and many did. But producing vaccines for large-scale use demanded far more substantial institutional resources and different skills. Many of the physician-innovators who established new institutions to produce sera and vaccines acquired those skills in Berlin or Paris.

In 1894 both Roux in Paris and Behring in Berlin announced that they had succeeded in producing a serum for treating (not preventing) diphtheria. While in both countries the result was public clamour and demand, production and distribution of sera and vaccines was organized quite differently in the two countries.

In Germany a commercial mode of production was soon established. In 1894 Behring left Berlin to become professor in Halle, and a year later in Marburg. By this time he had already begun discussions with the firm of Meister, Lucius and Bruning (later known as Farbwerke Hoechst), who agreed to finance his research in exchange for the right to produce and distribute the serum. However, they soon faced competition from another firm, Schering, which had developed a serum in collaboration with a scientist named Aronson attached to the Berlin veterinary school. Their competing products were available for purchase through licensed pharmacies, and each firm was scathingly critical of the other's product. In 1901 Behring was awarded the first Nobel Prize in Physiology or Medicine. He used the prize money as start-up capital, and in 1904 his company, Behringwerke, also began producing diphtheria serum. Soon a number of competing commercial sera were available for purchase in Germany. The state encouraged the alliances between research and industry that made this possible, but gradually became concerned that some products might be substandard. After all, anyone could in principle make diphtheria serum on the basis of published results, and the likelihood of profits might well tempt some unscrupulous entrants into the field, with potential risks to people's health.

In France, where the Pasteur Institute had a monopoly on serum production, these concerns did not arise. Thanks to huge contributions from the general public, from local communities and from the state, the Institute was able to expand production. Subscribers expected that the serum would be available at no cost to those who needed it but could not afford to pay, and this is what happened. When demand began to outstrip the Institute's ability to manufacture the serum, local centres of production emerged, mostly based in university medical faculties. In Bordeaux, for example, a professor who had been trained by Roux worked with the city authorities in setting up a production facility. People diagnosed by a physician as having diphtheria would be eligible for treatment. The serum was above all an instrument for protecting the health of the community, and unlike in Germany there was little commercial interest. But it also had another function.

For a colonial power such as France, transfer of these new public health technologies became an integral part of state policy. Though not a state institution, the Pasteur Institute had a distinctly 'imperial' mission. Support from the state was based on the hope that the Institute would help restore the country's prestige, badly damaged by defeat in the Franco–Prussian war. Though using bacteriological science to protect the health of French colonists was part of the Institute's mission, other strategic interests were also involved. From its very beginnings, the Pasteur Institute had planned to set up 'scientific colonies', or '*filiales*', which would propagate the Pasteurian doctrine and initiate local research, especially in 'exposed tropical countries'. This is what happened, and the Institute's policies led to the establishment of a worldwide network of bacteriological centres.

Alexandre Yersin was dispatched to Hong Kong, to investigate an epidemic of bubonic plague. There he succeeded in identifying the pathogen that causes the disease. (So, simultaneously, did Kitasato Shibasaburo, who had studied with Koch and Behring, and had established the Japanese Institute for the Study of Infectious Diseases a few years earlier.) Yersin returned to Paris and, working with Roux, Calmette and Borrle, prepared the first anti-bubonic plague serum. Setting off yet again, Yersin established a laboratory in French Indochina to produce the serum: a laboratory that later became a branch of the Pasteur Institute. Other Pasteur institutes followed, often established at the initiative of local governments – in Tunis, Senegal, Madagascar and elsewhere. Other initiatives failed, as a result of lack of political commitment or bureaucratic resistance.

Waldemar Haffkine went to India to test his cholera vaccine. With help from the British ambassador in Paris, who was a former viceroy of India, he obtained permission to do so. Travelling through the country for many months, he vaccinated thousands of people. Inevitably he faced numerous difficulties, both technical (ensuring adequate supplies of potent vaccine) and bureaucratic. Haffkine hoped to improve the conduct and reliability of his trials through use of a control group. Indeed he seems to have been one of the first to plan a trial using a control group – something that later became standard practice. But because the government insisted that all vaccinations should be voluntary, this was ultimately not possible. By mid-1896 he had decided that protection was achieved after five days but lasted for no longer than fourteen months. The work took its toll, however. Haffkine became sick from malaria and from overwork and was obliged to return to Europe to recuperate. Meanwhile, his work evoked so much interest in India that when an epidemic of plague broke out in Bombay, the governor invited Haffkine to Bombay to work on producing a plague vaccine. He accepted the challenge and managed to do so. The laboratory in which he worked (and then directed), first known as the Plague Research Laboratory, was subsequently renamed the Haffkine Institute.

Later historians have found a pattern in the diffusion of Pasteurian practices. New institutes typically began by offering treatments for rabies, sometimes combined with a laboratory for producing vaccine and diphtheria serum. Administrative structures varied, some being more and others less independent of decisions taken in Paris. Gradually, the system evolved. After the First World War, local initiatives to set up a Pasteur institute not only needed approval from Paris, but had to supply their own funding and to submit their choice of director to Paris.

Ties with the Pasteur Institute played an important role in the beginnings of vaccine production in many countries. Mexican president Porfirio Díaz had sent his personal physician to learn the new science in Paris, and when an Instituto Bacteriólogico Nacional was established in 1905 it developed close ties with the Pasteur Institute. Like similar institutes elsewhere, this institute combined basic bacteriological research with the production of vaccines and sera. After a decade of revolutionary unrest and political transformation the institute was renamed Instituto de Higiene, and then developed close ties with the Rockefeller Foundation. In Canada, Dr John G. FitzGerald, who had studied at the Pasteur Institutes in Paris and Brussels (as well as at the University of Freiburg), set up a laboratory in a stable building in Toronto in 1913. Fitzgerald was determined to provide his native country with the new tools of bacteriology at an affordable price. Within a few months, the University of Toronto had agreed to work with him, and the 'Antitoxin Laboratory', later the Connaught Laboratory, was established in the basement of the medical faculty building. The Connaught Laboratory produced diphtheria antitoxin, which it sold at a fraction of the cost of serum imported from the USA.

Like their French equivalents, British colonial civil servants also had to deal with public health problems in the areas they administered. To tackle disease in the huge territory of British India, in the last years of the nineteenth century and the first years of the twentieth public health institutions were set up across the country to do research and to develop and produce sera against cholera, rabies, tetanus, diphtheria, smallpox and typhoid. They included the King Institute of Preventive Medicine in Madras (now known as Chennai), the Haffkine Institute in Bombay (now Mumbai), the Central Research Institute Kasauli in 1905 and the Pasteur Institute of India at Coonoor. The CRI Kasauli and the Haffkine Institute were among the country's major vaccine and sera producers in the pre-independence period, with the former responsible for producing typhoid vaccine to be given to Indian troops fighting in the Middle East during the First World War. By 1930 there were around fifteen such state-sponsored institutions in the different provinces of British India, as well as a few private companies also making sera and vaccines.

As the value of the new sera and vaccines in preventing the spread of infectious disease found growing acceptance, production and provision became a legitimate element of public health policy. Some smaller European states soon equipped their public health laboratories to produce diphtheria serum: the Danish Statens Serum Institut (State Serum Institute or SSI) started work in 1902, and a Swedish institute (SBL) in 1909. In the Netherlands, while politicians debated the need for a central public health laboratory, in 1895 production of diphtheria antitoxin began in a private institution, the Bacterio-therapeutisch Instituut. In subsequent years it began to produce a variety of sera and vaccines, including against tetanus and rabies, some of which were exported to the Dutch colonies. Problems in meeting national needs during the First World War, coupled with political anxieties regarding security of supply and a sense of government responsibility, led the Dutch government to take over the institute in 1919, when it became the Rijks-serologisch Instituut.

In the United States, production of diphtheria serum began in the laboratory of the New York municipal department of health.

William H. Park, its German-trained chief bacteriologist, was soon able to produce it in accordance with instructions sent to him from Europe. As early as 1895, antitoxin was being produced for sale, the proceeds being used to purchase new laboratory equipment and to supply the antitoxin free in New York. Philadelphia was keen to follow the New York example. A small quantity of antitoxin was purchased from Behring while a facility (shared with the University of Pennsylvania) was being constructed. In fact the scale of production soon proved inadequate to the city's needs, and it was obliged to turn to the New York laboratory for additional supplies. However, in the United States public health departments did not have a monopoly on serum production for very long. The Philadelphia laboratory's first director became disenchanted with the funds the city would provide, resigned, and joined a local drug company that wanted to move into this new serum business. The New York laboratory, undoubted leader in the U.S., was quite willing to share its knowledge of production technology with others, irrespective of the public or private interests they represented. Commercial drug companies, including Mulford and Parke Davis, set about taking the lead from the municipal laboratories. Business historian Jonathan Liebenau described the strategy the budding vaccine industry followed. First companies learned what they could from the public health institutes. Then they tempted staff away. Then they set about discrediting public-sector vaccine and serum production, using two arguments: 'The first was that the municipal facilities were inadequate, and the second was that the government should not interfere with commercial enterprise by undercutting the commercial market.'[7] Liebenau argues that the public health laboratories' early success actually carried the seeds of their subsequent decline. The public officials on whom they depended for their funding were responsive to the arguments made by the commercial industry. The result was that by the time of the First World War there were at least half a dozen manufacturers of typhoid vaccine active in the U.S. market.

Regulation, Standardization and Proof

Turning basic discoveries in bacteriology into effective tools for combatting diphtheria, tuberculosis, typhoid and cholera involved creating institutions able to produce and distribute them in large quantities. Reduced to its bare bones, serum and vaccine production at the dawn of the twentieth century had two crucial steps. The first was essentially scientific. The pathogen had to be identified and isolated, generally from the bodily fluids of an infected person. In the second step, which was essentially technological, the pathogen had to be cultured, attenuated or inactivated, and the whole process had to be scaled up. As demand grew, so the number of organizations producing them multiplied. How could anyone be sure that everything being produced would protect people rather than actually making them sick? For governments increasingly committed to intervening in the interests of citizens' health and well-being, this question began to loom large. Both French and German authorities took steps in this direction. In France the responsibility was delegated to professional inspectors, who were required only to assess the adequacy of the facilities in which sera were being produced. They were not expected to test the quality of what was produced. Heads of the laboratories producing sera and vaccines, and the inspectors responsible for ensuring the standard of the facilities, had similar backgrounds. Most had been trained at the Pasteur Institute or were associated with it in some way. As historian Volker Hess points out, this made the Institute responsible not only for its own production, but also for the oversight of any potential competitors.[8] In Germany, production was based on a competitive market. Since any charlatan might set himself up as a serum producer, a far more rigorous approach was established. The state would have to find ways of regulating the quality of the substances being sold to the public as sera and vaccines. These steps – the regulatory processes – had quite distinct dynamics under state, and under market-oriented, systems of production.

In Germany a system of state control was established in the 1890s, regulating production and distribution processes as well as where and how the public could obtain serum. Companies wishing to produce serum for sale had first to apply for permission to produce it. They were then obliged to appoint a medical official, who reported to the state. In 1896 a new institute for Serum Testing and Research (Institut für Serumforschung und Serumprüfung) was set up in Berlin, with Paul Ehrlich (Behring's one-time colleague) as its director. All producers had to send a sample of every large batch of diphtheria antitoxin serum to Ehrlich's institute for testing. There the serum was mixed with toxin, in a ratio so that their effects cancelled each other out when injected into a guinea pig. But as there was a large margin of uncertainty in assessing whether symptoms of illness were present, Ehrlich established an unambiguous target: the death of the animal. The mixture was to be such that the test animal would die after exactly four days. If it died earlier, the serum was too weak and was rejected. Once a batch was approved, a certificate was issued and the medical official could release that batch of serum. Ehrlich's method enabled sera of standard potency to be prepared. This was vitally important in mass inoculation programmes. A memoir Ehrlich published in 1897, 'The Potency Estimation of Diphtheria Antiserum and its Theoretical Base', is often taken to mark the birth of biological standardization.

Though Ehrlich's procedure was complex and difficult to follow, its importance was recognized. In London, where Ehrlich lectured on his method of testing in 1900, Burroughs Wellcome had been producing serum since 1895. The company was well aware of the importance of ensuring the quality of its product. In 1903 the physiologist Henry Dale went to spend some months studying with Ehrlich before returning to London to join the staff of the company's Physiological Research Laboratories. However, the British government, unlike its German counterpart, was reluctant to get involved. Diphtheria still claimed thousands of lives at the end of the nineteenth century, and Burroughs Wellcome was only one of a number of manufacturers offering serum for sale in Britain. Nevertheless, unwilling to interfere with free trading practices, the British government moved slowly and reluctantly towards any kind of regulation. Even in the 1920s the British government was still unwilling to supply diphtheria serum or to recommend its general use, or to impose any kind of regulation on companies supplying it. British doctors wishing to vaccinate their patients had no guidance on which they could rely regarding the quality of competing products.

Their German colleagues were more fortunate. Though the Prussian state was not involved in producing serum, leaving this to private drug companies, it did regulate both who was permitted to produce serum, and the quality of what they produced. Unlike their British counterparts, German doctors and the parents of children to be treated could be confident that the serum employed was both safe and effective. Prussian administrative practices were important both for development of techniques of biological standardization and for development of the practice of regulatory oversight.

In addition to these technical and administrative procedures, the 1920s also saw the emergence of yet another set of techniques with major importance for the future of mass vaccination. While diphtheria serum had been used in treatment, the recovery of a patient offered a convincing demonstration that it worked. With technologies of prevention, matters are different. There is no immediate or obvious proof of their effectiveness. Data have to be assembled, possibly from large numbers of people, and have to be analysed and interpreted. Since BCG was not intended to cure tuberculosis, it was not possible to use a patient's recovery as an indicator of efficacy. How could people be convinced that it actually protected them against infection? What kind of evidence would carry sufficient authority, and how could it be collected?

In the 1920s the Pasteur Institute, which had a monopoly, was producing BCG and providing it to medical practitioners throughout France. Any doctor or midwife in the country could contact the Institute and ask for the three doses for a named baby. They would be asked to supply clinical data on the child in the following years. By December 1926 almost twenty thousand infants had received BCG. Thanks to its monopoly, the Pasteur Institute was able to ensure a standardized and stable product. Because the vaccine was perishable, it retained its potency for only a few days, so that efficient production and distribution were essential. It would be impossible supply it from Paris to areas beyond metropolitan France. So the Pasteur Institute delegated production to foreign laboratories, mobilizing in the first instance its own widespread international network.

Calmette had little interest in statistics. But even though medical statistics were then in their infancy, he was forced to acknowledge that in order to convince the profession that the vaccine worked he would need some statistical data. Specifically, he would have to compare vaccinated with unvaccinated children. In order to do this Calmette needed to know the expected rate of TB mortality among unvaccinated children. With the aid of a questionnaire sent to dispensaries around the country, he calculated a TB infant mortality rate of 24 per cent. In other words he concluded that 24 out of every one hundred babies who contracted tuberculosis would die of it within their first year. By contrast the mortality of children in the hospital who had been vaccinated was less than 1 per cent. For Calmette these numbers were proof enough of the vaccine's efficacy. It could be used with confidence. Outside France, however, not everyone was convinced by Calmette's statistics. Ideas of evidence, what it took to prove convincingly that something worked, were changing.

Data from all the BCG users were collected and collated in Paris, and in 1927–8 the statistical analysis was made available throughout the world. These statistics, which for Calmette constituted proof of the vaccine's effectiveness, and which in France benefited from the status of the Institute, were subjected to a barrage of international criticism. Why had further tests on the children not been done? How did conclusions based on the simple fact that the children appeared healthy after 24 months fit with the poor response to the tuberculin test for tuberculosis immunity? Perhaps the problem was the oral administration? The Scandinavians had started injecting the vaccine, whereas the French were still administering it orally. What was the correct baseline: the mortality rate to be expected in the absence of vaccination? Calmette had estimated a tuberculosis-related mortality rate among unvaccinated children of 24 per cent, whereas a study in Copenhagen had found it to be only around 5 per cent. From London, Major Greenwood, a leading figure in the new field of epidemiology, questioned the comparability of the vaccinated and unvaccinated children in Calmette's work. Greenwood doubted that the sample was large enough for any reliable conclusions to be reached. In 1928 the question of whether BCG worked, and the kind of data needed to establish its efficacy, was taken up by the League of Nations Health Organization. The expert panel that was set up largely endorsed Greenwood's critique, to the effect that the sampling was unclear. Not only was it unclear how the children to be vaccinated had been selected, but since no autopsies had been carried out it was impossible to know which deaths were actually due to TB. The experts insisted that in order to reach statistically reliable conclusions it was essential to work with a control group: that is, with groups of vaccinated and unvaccinated children that in other relevant respects were comparable.

Ideas of a control group and randomization were not wholly new. Haffkine had wanted to work with a control group, though he had been unable to do so for political reasons. Johannes Fibiger, a Danish physician–researcher, had greater success in this respect. When he returned to Copenhagen after studying with Koch and Behring in Berlin, Fibiger began research on diphtheria. In 1896, working as a junior hospital doctor, he convinced his superiors that published studies showing the efficacy of serum treatment for diphtheria were unreliable. In 1896 and 1897 Fibiger carried out the first randomized trial. Whether or not patients with diphtheria received the serum treatment or not was made to depend on the day they were admitted to the hospital. Of the roughly one thousand patients admitted in the year, about half were excluded for one reason or another. The other five hundred or so were allocated to the 'study', or to the 'control' arm of the trial by alternating from day to day. The results of the study, which showed the serum treatment to be effective, were published in 1898. However, because they were published in Danish, which few people outside Denmark could read, these results attracted little attention internationally. It was only thirty years later, in the 1920s, that the idea that convincing evidence required randomization and a control group began to gain support. (In the late 1930s it was still common practice for new treatments to be introduced on the basis of no more than the conviction of an eminent professor in a leading medical faculty, probably based on what he had seen in a few of his patients.)

Despite his distaste for statistics, Calmette had to respond if his vaccine was to be widely used. The vaccine's reputation was not helped by the deaths of 76 German babies, said to be due to their BCG vaccinations. Calmette's difficulty was that the international group of statistical experts was demanding use of a control group and randomization, but it would be impossible to conduct such a study in France because family doctors would object. Calmette therefore turned to Algiers, where a branch of the Pasteur Institute was already producing and distributing BCG. The city had a well-organized system for collecting demographic data, and the Muslim population of its poorest and most densely populated areas suffered very high rates of deaths from TB. These were perfect conditions for the randomized trial that Calmette wanted.

In the course of the first two or three decades of the century, elements of a system for developing and producing biological tools (sera and vaccines) for protecting public health were starting

to fall into place. Techniques for isolating, identifying and cultivating bacilli were becoming more and more sophisticated. But
vaccine production was never only a matter of bacteriological *science*. Institutions to produce them, statistical methods, regulatory
regimes, biological standards, systems for safely transporting and
administering these (often fragile) materials: all of these were no
less vital. The form institutions and practices took differed from
place to place. In many countries production facilities were established by national or local governments, often combining public
health research with serum production. Elsewhere, as in Prussia,
production was in the hands of private companies. These two models
were carried far afield, often by physicians trained in bacteriology
in Berlin or Paris, and sometimes supported by political interests
(whether imperial or nationalistic). Since biological tools lose their
potency over time, they are best produced as near to the site of
use as possible. Experience with diphtheria serum taught that dis-
persed production and use of these materials also required a system
of standardization and regulation if safety and potency were to be
ensured. Standardization and regulation fitted well with Prussian
administrative traditions, though the stringent regulatory system
developed there did not appeal to politicians everywhere. Thus we
see that whereas some governments assumed responsibility for producing the vaccines their public health systems required, others
limited their role to ensuring that vaccines produced commercially
were of good quality so that people could have confidence in them.
Yet other governments were reluctant to intervene in any way at
all. Thus the British government delayed taking any responsibility
for regulatory oversight until the late 1920s. With the emergence
of the new discipline of epidemiology came profound changes in
the standards that evidence for the efficacy of a prophylactic tool
would have to meet.

Edward Jenner had pointed the way and Louis Pasteur had
cleared it. As techniques were improved, attention turned from the
relatively obscure diseases, such as anthrax and rabies, on which
Pasteur had first focused, to diseases of major public health concern.
There were many of these at the start of the twentieth century, not
only smallpox, but typhoid, diphtheria, cholera, tuberculosis, plague
and yellow fever. All of these were major threats, claiming large
numbers of lives. Moreover, quarantine, which for decades had been

a crucial component of public health, had critical disadvantages in an era of rapidly expanding trade. It not only disrupted international commerce but it could lead to political frictions between nations. The diffusion of vaccine technology (both process and product) from Paris and Berlin around 1900 was complex, propelled by a number of interests and considerations. In addition to the humanitarian aspect there were various political interests, ranging from ensuring the functioning and profitability of the colonies, to the exercise of civic responsibilities. And there was always a commercial interest, more or less overt, and varying in its significance from country to country. It is almost impossible to disentangle these, since vaccines have always been simultaneously tools for the relief or prevention of suffering, tools of control, and potentially profitable commodities. What is clear, however, is that the burden of disease – public health need – was the principal influence on where bacteriologists turned their attention. The diseases against which sera and vaccines were sought were among those causing the greatest suffering and death.

THREE

TECHNOLOGIES:
VIRAL CHALLENGES

Bacteriology was moving forwards rapidly in the first years of the twentieth century and had already provided medicine with some important new tools in its fight against infectious disease. One was a new treatment for syphilis. After a long series of painstaking experiments, in 1909 Paul Ehrlich had found an organic compound of arsenic that would destroy its cause, a kind of bacterium known as a spirochaete. Ehrlich's anti-syphilitic drug, which he thought of as a 'magic bullet', was marketed by Hoechst AG under the name Salvarsan. There were vaccines against rabies and diphtheria, and a promising typhoid vaccine. In many European countries institutions equipped to produce these new public health tools had been established, some attached to public health departments, some to commercial businesses. Then, in the summer of 1914, Europe was thrown into bloody turmoil. The war triggered by the assassination of Archduke Franz Ferdinand, heir to the Hapsburg throne, and Austro-Hungary's subsequent declaration of war on Serbia, was to last more than four years. The death toll among both civilians and armed forces was horrendous. Millions died, not only from shelling and from poison gas attacks, but also from disease. The filth and the lack of sanitation with which soldiers fighting in muddy trenches had to contend meant that outbreaks of diseases such as typhoid and typhus were a constant threat. It was in this context, in which soldiers' health was constantly challenged, that Wright and Leishman's typhoid vaccine proved itself. Of the British soldiers going off to fight on the front, 97 per cent were vaccinated, and deaths from typhoid among British combatants were far fewer than they had been in previous campaigns.

The Versailles negotiations that followed the end of the First World War changed the map of Europe and the Middle East. The old empires, Austro-Hungarian and Ottoman, but also (as a result of the Russian Revolution) Russian, vanished, and new states were born. In 1920 a League of Nations was established, with headquarters in Geneva, with a mandate principally to maintain world peace and resolve international disputes. In much of Europe living conditions had deteriorated dramatically, and public health, infectious disease control in particular, was receiving growing attention. The League of Nations made health one of its concerns, and established a permanent Health Bureau as well as various advisory bodies. It was here that the adequacy of Calmette's BCG data was later to be questioned. The League's health organization soon embarked on ambitious international campaigns. It hoped, for example, to eliminate the mosquitoes that caused malaria and yellow fever.

Internationally, the Rockefeller Foundation also played a key role. It provided financial support to the League of Nations Health Organization. It organized large-scale population health surveys and hookworm and yellow fever eradication programmes in much of Latin America. It was also active in Central Europe. Working through its International Health Board, the Foundation set out to help the new states that had emerged from the wreckage of the old empires to develop effective public health systems. Social stability, democracy and good health went together, as far as the Foundation was concerned, so that it was unwilling to provide any assistance to the Soviet Union. The Rockefeller Foundation carried out a series of missions intended to assess possibilities for establishing new institutes of hygiene and training programmes in public health modelled on the one at Johns Hopkins University in the United States. The experts sent as advisers to fledgling ministries of health were often frustrated by the administrative traditions that persisted in many new countries as a legacy of their Austro-Hungarian or Ottoman heritage.

In Britain a Ministry of Health was established in 1919. The wartime work of the Medical Research Committee, organizing and coordinating medical research, was put on a permanent basis in a new Medical Research Council. With growing political attention to public health, welfare and medical research, other countries began to take similar steps. Persia's minister of foreign affairs, who was serving as the head of his country's delegation to the 1919 Versailles

Peace Conference, used the opportunity of his visit to contact the Pasteur Institute. He invited the French bacteriologists to help his government tackle the country's public health problems by establishing an affiliated institute in Persia. The French were very willing, since this fitted precisely with the Institute's mission, and in 1920 a French bacteriologist left for Teheran.

'Filterable Viruses'

As the war was ending an influenza epidemic of unprecedented severity swept the globe. The symptoms of influenza had been known for hundreds of years: high temperature, sore throat, tiredness, headache, aching limbs, coughing. Generally, victims recovered after suffering for a few days. But the influenza that struck in 1918 was different. Unlike earlier epidemics, it didn't affect principally the young and the elderly: it attacked adults in the prime of life, the group at greatest risk being those aged twenty to forty. Combat was brought to a standstill in places as soldiers succumbed. It arrived in two waves, the first (in spring 1918) less virulent than the second (in the autumn). It came to be known as the 'Spanish flu' though it didn't originate there and had no particular association with Spain. Subsequent estimates of the death toll wrought by the epidemic range from twenty million to a hundred million people, spread over the whole planet. In Britain alone, some 200,000 people died. It was the deaths of hundreds of thousands of its citizens that led the Persian government to seek help from the Pasteur Institute. Whatever its past successes, in 1918 the new science was confronted with a challenge that it was unable to meet.

No one understood why influenza had suddenly become so much more serious. The common view among medical scientists was that influenza was caused by a bacterial agent known as Pfeiffer's bacillus. Richard Pfeiffer, a student and then colleague of Robert Koch, made many important discoveries in bacteriology and immunology. In 1892 he had isolated a bacillus from the noses of patients suffering an attack of flu. He called it *Bacillus influenzae*, though it was more commonly known as Pfeiffer's bacillus (and today as *Haemophilus influenzae*). Hoping to combat the Spanish flu epidemic, scientists set about isolating the bacillus in order to produce a vaccine in the same manner as previous vaccines had been prepared. Unfortunately, in many flu victims there was no sign of the bacillus. Vaccines were prepared from various bacteria linked with respiratory diseases, including Pfeiffer's bacillus and pneumococcus, but none of them offered any protection against the influenza. As bacteriology's unexpected impotence in the face of the pandemic became clear, fearful people clutched at any straw. Purveyors of patent medicines, like the Alan Krumwiede character in *Contagion*, were more than happy to hold out such straws. At the same time some scientists were starting to think that this bacillus might not, in fact, be the cause of influenza. What else could be the cause? Insight into what it might be came, slowly and indirectly, from a quite different field of biological research.

In the course of the nineteenth century tobacco had become a commercially important crop, so that a late nineteenth-century outbreak of disease among tobacco plants had major economic consequences. What came to be known as tobacco mosaic disease was identified in Wageningen, in the Netherlands, in the 1880s. It was shown to be transmissible from one plant to another, though there was considerable uncertainty as to its cause. Tobacco crops in Russia had also been affected, and Dmitri Ivanovsky was sent to investigate. His major contribution, in 1892, was to show that the agent that caused the disease passed through the extremely fine filters that had been developed in order to collect bacteria – though Ivanovsky nevertheless believed the pathogen was a bacterium. The problem was then picked up by the Dutch bacteriologist Martinus Beijerinck, who had been intrigued by the uncertainties of the earlier Dutch research. Beijerinck too found that the causative agent couldn't be collected with the porcelain filters that retained bacteria. An inspired researcher, he was able to establish that it multiplied only in living tissue. Standard tools of bacteriological investigation were of little use, since this pathogen could neither be cultivated *in vitro*, nor viewed under the microscope. Drawing on his knowledge of chemistry, Beijerinck became convinced that what he was dealing with was not a bacterium at all, but something far simpler. He conjectured that it was nothing more than a large molecule that – somehow – was able to reproduce itself, though only in living tissue. Beijerinck called it the tobacco mosaic 'virus', from the Latin word meaning a poison or venom. The idea that a plant disease could be caused by a mere molecule seemed absurd, no more than a flight of fancy, to most of Beijerinck's contemporaries. However, around the start of the twentieth century a number of other pathogens (including that causing foot and mouth disease among cattle) that also passed through bacteriologists' filters were found. The term 'virus' stuck. The new organisms became known as 'filterable viruses', and in the early years of the twentieth century others were found, mainly as a result of studying diseases of animals, especially poultry.

In 1901 Eugenio Centanni, professor of pathology in Ferrara, demonstrated the filterability of the agent causing fowl plague. It became a focus for much subsequent research into the nature of viruses. Though researchers were anxious to find a way of cultivating viruses that avoided the need for animals, no artificial media had worked. Centanni went on to make another discovery that would later prove of great importance for vaccine production. He injected the fowl plague virus into fertilized hen's eggs and found that it killed the embryo and itself survived, though without multiplying. Centanni was unsure as to the nature of the substance he had isolated. Was it a living organism, a complex chemical molecule or something in between? Francesco Sanfelice at the University of Modena showed that the agent causing fowl pox behaved as a protein – though one that, mysteriously, was able to reproduce itself within a living cell. Sanfelice's view seems to have been close to what his contemporaries envisaged the cause of tobacco mosaic disease to be. However, because the one studied diseases in animals and the other diseases in plants they were unaware of each other's work. There was as yet no discipline of 'virology' in which researchers studying human, animal and plant viruses – or those infecting bacteria, which were later to prove of enormous importance for the emergence of molecular biology – read each other's work and interacted.

A disease being intensively studied at this time was yellow fever. Decades earlier, the Cuban physician Carlos Finlay had conjectured that it was carried by mosquitoes. For years, yellow fever prevention had emphasized mosquito control, and with considerable success. However, attempts to isolate the infectious agent carried by the mosquitoes had all failed. In 1902 a United States Army commission, investigating yellow fever in Cuba, concluded that it too was caused by a 'filterable virus'. This was the first disease of humans attributed to infection by this new kind of entity. Thereafter, both the Rockefeller Foundation's West Africa Yellow Fever Commission, based in Nigeria, and the Pasteur Institute in Senegal set about trying to isolate the virus. In 1927 both groups succeeded, though at a price. In both laboratories some of the researchers caught yellow fever and died. Once the virus had been identified researchers could investigate its whereabouts and the ways in which it was transmitted. It was found to be common in a number of species of monkey, in both Africa and Latin America. Both the monkeys and human communities living in close proximity to them were found to have developed antibodies to the virus. And so far as its mode of transmission was concerned, Carlos Finlay had been right. His conjecture that it was carried by mosquitoes was borne out.

Prior to the 1918 epidemic, influenza had been viewed as one of the normal risks of modern city life. But after 1918 its significance had changed. 'When will it turn so deadly again?' is a question as salient today as it was then. There was heightened popular awareness of the disease, and it ranked high among the complaints with which patients visited their GP in the 1920s. Although at this time relatively few people died directly of influenza, an infection could lead to pneumonia. This was far more serious, and many people died as a result of pneumonia that followed a bout of flu. Despite growing speculation that influenza might be caused by a virus, there was little direct evidence that this was in fact so. The only investigator who had apparently succeeded in infecting people (and monkeys) with a pathogenic agent that passed through a filter (that is, a virus) was Charles Nicolle at the Pasteur Institute in Tunis. However, there had only been two or three humans in his study, and though the work was presented at the French Academy of Science, it did not have much impact. In Britain the new Medical Research Council (MRC) devoted particular attention to research on viruses. The 1918 Spanish flu epidemic, 'the greatest pandemic since the Black Death', was a useful referent when it came to gathering political support for the plan. Evidence was starting to accumulate, and by the early 1920s more and more scientists were convinced that influenza was indeed caused by a virus.

In the course of the 1930s, though scientists continued to debate whether viruses should be regarded as living organisms or as mere chemicals, knowledge of them was growing. In 1935 the American biochemist Wendell Stanley crystallized a protein that he claimed had the properties of tobacco mosaic virus (though his findings were subsequently questioned). Gradually scientists studying viral diseases of plants, animals and humans were starting to interact and a discipline of virology was beginning to take shape. There was a growing consensus that viruses consist only of proteins combined with some kind of genetic material. As has so often been the case in science, developments were greatly facilitated by the development of new instruments. Although viruses were too small to be seen with a light microscope, in the 1930s development of a new kind of microscope, which uses a beam of electrons instead of visible light, literally threw new light on them.

If vaccines against viral diseases such as influenza and yellow fever were to be developed, the standard steps used in preparing bacterial vaccines – isolation, cultivation and attenuation/inactivation of the pathogen – would have to be adapted. After all, the viruses wouldn't grow in test tubes, and little was known as to how they could best be attenuated or inactivated. In 1931 Alice Woodruff and Ernest Goodpasture, at Vanderbilt University, perfected the method of inoculating fertilized eggs that Centanni had tried out thirty years previously. They were able to show that embryonic cells of the chick's chorio-allantoic membrane (the avian equivalent of a placenta) provided an excellent medium for the cultivation of viruses. A smallpox vaccine prepared in chick embryos was just as effective as one prepared in calves. It had the great advantage of avoiding the risk of bacterial contamination that use of a live animal could entail. The use of fertilized hen's eggs was to prove invaluable for vaccine production.

Developing an Influenza Vaccine

At the start of the 1930s research on influenza vaccine was moving forwards slowly, as the virus that caused it had still not been isolated. In 1933 scientists at the National Institute for Medical Research in London took mucus from the noses or throats of influenza-infected people and squirted it into the noses of ferrets (animals that were widely used in veterinary research). If an animal developed the symptoms of human influenza its lung tissue would be dried, ground, filtered and used to inoculate another animal. By 1935 these London-based researchers, as well as Thomas Rivers in the USA and Frank MacFarlane Burnet in Australia, had established not only that influenza was caused by a virus, but also that ferrets that had been infected were resistant to reinfection. The first step towards development of a vaccine had been taken, and in the late 1930s the first influenza vaccine trials began. The outbreak of the Second World War gave new impetus to the search for an effective vaccine, just as the First World War had added urgency to the development of typhoid vaccine. Large concentrations of soldiers provide a perfect breeding ground for infectious diseases, and memories of the 1918 epidemic were still vivid.

Three important developments took place in the early 1940s. At the University of Melbourne, MacFarlane Burnet (who was to win the Nobel Prize in 1960) showed that the flu virus would grow well in fertilized hen's eggs. In New York George Hirst, working at the Rockefeller Institute, found that fluid taken from infected chick embryos caused red blood cells to form clumps. It didn't make any difference if the blood cells came from chicks or from humans. This discovery formed the basis of the 'haemagglutination test', which could be used to establish the quantity of virus in a sample. These two techniques greatly facilitated influenza vaccine development. On the other hand, complicating matters was the discovery that there exist more than one type of influenza virus, and that immunity to one didn't confer immunity to another. A strain isolated by Thomas Francis at the University of Michigan became 'influenza B', while that isolated earlier in London (later shown to be closely related to avian viruses such as fowl plague) became 'influenza A'. Making matters still more complicated, it appeared that there are various strains of each type. What would have to be included in a vaccine for it to be effective?

As it prepared to enter the war, the United States intensified its efforts in the influenza field. In 1941 the Armed Forces created a Commission on Influenza, containing a number of the country's leading virologists and influenza vaccine researchers. Thomas Francis chaired the commission, which made development of an effective vaccine a major priority. Though most American researchers in the field thought that only an attenuated virus vaccine would work, Francis thought otherwise. Assisted by an enthusiastic young New Yorker named Jonas Salk, Francis set about developing an inactivated vaccine, first using ultraviolet light to kill the virus, and then chemical agents. By 1942, a formalin-inactivated vaccine containing type B virus and a number of type A strains was ready for testing, and by 1945 a commercially produced vaccine could be given to all soldiers. It was very effective. At first. But then, strangely, it began to fail. In a 1947 epidemic the vaccine was found to provide no protection whatever. What was going on? Researchers couldn't agree as to whether the strains found in 1947 were simply new sub-types of type A virus, or whether something more complex and worrying was going on. MacFarlane Burnet thought the virus was mutating, and there were growing doubts among influenza researchers as to the feasibility of long-term protection. In 1949 a further complication arose when a third type of influenza virus was found to infect dogs and pigs (though relatively rarely humans). It was designated influenza type C. A World Influenza Centre was established at the National Institute for Medical Research in London, and research on the virus, its properties, its mutations and on the effectiveness of different kinds of vaccine continued. We'll return to the influenza virus in the next chapter.

Jonas Salk, who had assisted Thomas Francis with his work on inactivated influenza vaccine, would soon become world famous for a different achievement in the fight against viral diseases.

Polio: A False Start

In 1932 Franklin Roosevelt became president of the United States. A decade earlier, Roosevelt, a wealthy and promising New York lawyer, had been stricken by the disease commonly known as infantile paralysis. Having lost the use of his lower limbs as a result, Roosevelt was confined to a wheelchair.

'Infantile paralysis', or poliomyelitis, was all too familiar, and widely feared in the United States. In 1916 New York had been struck by an epidemic which had led to nine thousand cases and more than 2,300 deaths. The city's Department of Health had tried to deal with it by means of the quarantine and sanitation campaigns that had been effective with other epidemics. They didn't work because, unlike most of the diseases that had plagued the nineteenth century, this was not a poverty-related disease. It didn't strike poor neighbourhoods with greatest severity. Though it was often known as 'infantile paralysis', it was actually not infants but older children and young adults who were most likely to be severely stricken. In the interwar years no disease could compare with poliomyelitis for the terror it evoked among parents, especially in the United States. Epidemics struck in the summer months. In many communities it was common to close swimming pools, beaches and playgrounds in order to limit possible cross-infection by children who might carry the virus but show no symptoms.

Polio was known to be caused by a virus. Karl Landsteiner, a Viennese physician–researcher who later became famous for his discovery of blood groups, had identified it earlier. What was not known was how the virus entered the body or how it reached the central nervous system and caused paralysis. Inspired by President Roosevelt's commitment to fighting the disease, scientists were gradually making progress. They were starting to understand that people infected with the virus excrete some of it, so that in places with poor sanitation some is very likely to find its way into the water people drink or use for cooking, washing or swimming. This was why children living in poor communities with poor sanitation could acquire a mild infection early on, and as a result become immune. Children in wealthy neighbourhoods enjoying the highest standards of hygiene would not have this immunity.

In studies using monkeys it was established that the virus infects the nerve cells in the spinal cord that provide stimuli to muscles, and which do not regenerate. Without these stimuli the muscles cease to function, and the patient could lose use of his or her limbs, or lose the ability to breath unaided.

As researchers began to understand what they thought was the mechanism of infection, hope of producing a vaccine grew. The problem for 1930s researchers, however, was that the polio virus appeared only to grow in nerve-cell tissue, and this was known to be very risky. Even the slightest impurities carried the risk that the culture could cause encephalitis. For this reason many leading virologists thought that it would never be possible to produce a safe polio vaccine. This didn't stop one or two researchers from trying. The consequences, in the 1930s, were disastrous. Maurice Brody at New York University School of Medicine made a formalin-inactivated vaccine that was tried out on hundreds of children. Other researchers, repeating his procedure, found that the virus wasn't wholly inactivated. In Philadelphia, Temple University's John Kolmer tried out an attenuated vaccine. A few children died and others contracted the disease as a result. Although MacFarlane Burnet had discovered that there was more than one type of polio virus a few years previously, it wasn't yet known how many there were, nor was it yet known how far immunity to one type conferred immunity to another. The time was not yet ripe. More had to be known before there was any hope of a polio vaccine that could responsibly be tried out on human volunteers.

The Aftermath of the Second World War: Reconstruction

The late 1940s and early 1950s were a time of shortage and reconstruction in much of the world, of populations weary, hungry and often homeless. In Europe, providing decent healthcare to the millions who had been left destitute, homeless or starving was high on any list of problems. In Britain the new Labour government, determined to make decent healthcare available to everyone, established the National Health Service. Moreover, the technological successes of the Second World War – the atomic bomb, radar, computing – inspired an increasingly technological vision of a better future. They inspired paranoia too, as fear of an imminent Cold War led to political obsession with the future control of atomic energy. More positively, some viewed technological advance as the source of wondrous improvements in what medicine would be able to accomplish. David Sarnoff, chairman of the Radio Corporation of America, imagined miniaturized electronic implants taking over the function of non-functioning organs. Visions like this played their part, but healthcare was moving in a new direction for another reason too. As scientists and technologists returned from war service new uses had to be found both for their skills and for the industrial capacity that had been tied up in the war effort. Some of the scientists and engineers returning to civilian life would find their way into the development of new medical technologies.

But many countries also faced an enormous effort of reconstruction. West European countries that had been occupied or annexed by Nazi Germany, once liberated, faced the challenge of reconstructing their institutions of government, of economic production and of research. In the Netherlands, for example, the Institute of Public Health (in Dutch RIV, later RIVM) had played a central role in the supply of vaccines since the 1930s. In the immediate post-war period, lack of facilities, space and manpower hindered efforts to produce the newer vaccines such as that against whooping cough (pertussis) that had recently been developed. In 1950 the Institute was reorganized, its tasks more clearly set out, and new staff appointed. By 1952 it had succeeded in producing a combination DPT (diphtheria-pertussis-tetanus) vaccine, and a new facility for smallpox vaccine had been constructed.

Elsewhere political turmoil and the need to rebuild institutions had different roots. In the Indian subcontinent the end of the Second World War was soon followed by the withdrawal of the British, and by independence and partition. In the field of medical science the British had done little to develop the kind of institutions an independent India (or an independent Pakistan) would require. As far as vaccine science and technology were concerned, the policies of the colonial state had failed to lay the foundation for a sustainable path for the development of vaccines. Only short-term research and production needs had been encouraged. Increased demand for vaccines and sera during the epidemics and the war, and the transfer of key staff to military service, had led to the old institutions being stripped of their research functions and had turned them into mere production units. There was a bare minimum of infrastructure, manpower and resources.

In 1948 the World Health Organization (WHO) was established as part of the United Nations system. Among the responsibilities it took over from the League of Nations Health Organization was standardization of biological products. There was a widespread feeling that much of the world's vaccine supply was not potent enough, or was unsafe. Many countries in which vaccines were being produced lacked any means of controlling their quality. Thus, soon after its establishment, the WHO created an Expert Committee on Biological Standardization, which was to set standards of quality for each vaccine, as well as other biological products used in healthcare. Not long afterwards the World Health Assembly, the WHO's 'parliament', recommended that nations should all adopt reference standards being set for the sterility, toxicity and potency of specific vaccines. Agreed testing procedures would have to be followed, and independent national control authorities would have to check that guidelines were being followed and that batches of vaccine were safe and sufficiently potent.

In the field of medical research, as in science generally, by the 1950s the centre of gravity had shifted. Leadership in science and technology had passed from Europe to the USA. Many leading scientists had fled Nazi persecution and found refuge in U.S. universities, while others were starting to flee the Communist regimes taking power in much of Eastern and Central Europe. Moreover, the undeniably successful organization of wartime science had partially mitigated long-standing mistrust of state interference. While before the war a private philanthropic institution (the Rockefeller Foundation) had been the main supporter of medical research in the United States, now the federal government was becoming increasingly involved. The National Institutes of Health (NIH) had been established in 1930, and in the 1940s its budget began to grow, rising sharply in the 1950s.

Polio Vaccines

In 1938 President Roosevelt and his friend and associate Basil O'Connor had created a National Foundation for Infantile Paralysis (later known as the 'March of Dimes') to raise money for polio research from the American public. A Scientific Advisory Committee chaired by Thomas Rivers had been established, and the Foundation was soon to play a key role in supporting development of a safe and effective polio vaccine. Pharmaceutical companies were also starting to interest themselves in viral vaccines. A central figure in this virus research, whose work led directly to the development of safe and effective polio vaccines, was Harvard professor John Enders.

Coming from a rich New England banking family, Enders had studied literature at Yale before abandoning an MA in philology to retrain in biology. In the late 1930s he was an assistant professor in Harvard Medical School's Department of Bacteriology and Immunology, and had begun to study the mumps virus. By 1948 he had succeeded in growing the virus in a tissue culture. Shortly thereafter, there being some culture (made from human embryonic skin and muscle tissue) left over, he thought he would put some polio virus into it, just on the off-chance. It grew – in non-nervous tissue. But that had been one strain only. However, other strains from other types worked too, and the embryo culture could be replaced by other sorts of non-nervous tissue cultures. The work was published in *Science* in January 1949, and thereafter interest in developing a vaccine grew rapidly. Frederick Robbins, who participated in this research, has explained just how crude, by today's standards, it had been. 'A bit of tissue was cut up into little bits that were placed in small flasks with nutrient fluid. The flasks were incubated at body temperature and approximately every four days the fluid was removed and replaced with fresh fluid.'[1] This replacement of the fluid was apparently innovative, though the work was by no means the result of a carefully planned research strategy! They'd had some polio virus in the freezer and Enders had suggested that they put some in the fluid to see what happened. They did not expect much since other investigators had failed to grow the virus other than in human nerve tissue. Their culture was made from the brains, muscle, kidney or intestine of aborted human foetuses. Later it was found that a culture made from monkey kidney tissue also worked well. While polio virus had only been grown in nerve cell tissue, a safe and effective polio vaccine had seemed unlikely. Now, suddenly, it was becoming feasible. In January 1949 the first publication announcing polio-virus cultivation in non-nerve cell culture appeared. From that time on, people from all over the world came to visit the Harvard laboratory, despite the fact that Enders had no personal interest in developing a polio vaccine.

Experience with influenza had taught that in order to make an effective vaccine, knowing whether more than one type of virus exists, and if so which ones are principally responsible for disease outbreaks, is crucial. By 1948 there was a feeling that there must be three types of polio virus. But this feeling wasn't enough to go on. More certainty was needed. The work that would have to be done, known as 'virus typing', was widely regarded as dull and boring and few researchers were willing to do it. Jonas Salk was one who was. In 1949, with support from the National Foundation/March of Dimes, he set to work. He needed a great many monkeys, since monkeys were the only animal known to be susceptible to all types of polio. Salk's work confirmed that there are indeed three types of polio virus (which came to be known as I, II and III). As knowledge of the polio virus accumulated, the issues that would have to be faced in producing a vaccine became clearer. First, immunity against one type doesn't mean immunity against another, and an effective vaccine would have to protect against all types. But there are also various strains of each type (though most strains had been found to belong to type I) and although any strain will generally protect against other strains of the same type, they differ somewhat in their properties. Most importantly, some strains of a given type are more virulent than others. Since the more virulent (and thus dangerous) a strain was, the better it was likely to be at stimulating production of antibodies, a difficult trade-off had to be made in deciding which strains to include in the vaccine.

Salk wanted to move on from his virus typing to development of a vaccine, and he hoped that the Foundation would provide him with the resources he would need. Sailing back to the USA from a polio congress in Copenhagen, in September 1951, Salk talked with O'Connor. Influenced by his earlier apprenticeship with Francis, Salk had decided to make a killed-virus vaccine, and on the voyage home he managed to convince O'Connor to back him. The Foundation's support flew in the teeth of opinion among virologists, most of whom, including John Enders, were convinced that a killed virus vaccine could not work. In order to produce a vaccine, Salk needed one strain from each of the three types. Types II and III were easy, but type I was the most common, and choosing a type I strain proved difficult. Salk eventually opted for the so-called Mahoney strain, which is particularly virulent and should therefore be particularly antigenic. He then had to decide on three crucial parameters: the temperature and time for inactivation, and the proportions of virus to the chemical (formalin) that would kill it. By early 1952 he was able to produce large quantities of killed virus, grown in monkey kidney culture. The product was then suspended in a mineral oil that would make it injectable and also serve as an adjuvant. Tested on monkeys it seemed to work. The next step that Salk took would today be regarded as wholly unethical. Packing some of the vaccine into his car, he tested it on children in the Watson Home for Crippled Children, near Pittsburgh. Everything went as he'd hoped, and the children developed antibodies. When other leading researchers heard about it they refused to be convinced by Salk's results. Nevertheless, by 1953 public pressure for a vaccine was such that the National Foundation decided that it couldn't wait any longer before starting a large-scale field trial. Thomas Francis at the University of Michigan was invited to direct the trial. He agreed, but only on the condition that it be a double-blind study:

that is, neither the people being vaccinated nor the investigators would know who was receiving the vaccine and who was receiving a placebo. Medical statistics, and standards of proof, had moved on since Calmette's time.

A lot of vaccine would be required for a trial of the size being planned, and six pharmaceutical companies were invited to produce it. Scaling up Salk's procedure in a reproducible and standard manner proved difficult, and the companies had problems producing vaccine that met all the safety requirements. But by March 1954 they had succeeded. In a three-month campaign that started the following month more than 440,000 children were given the vaccine and more than 200,000 a placebo. While the data from the trial were being analysed, Foundation officials were wrestling with a very different problem. If the vaccine was found to have worked there would be an instant demand for millions of doses. In order to have these ready on time, manufacturers would have to start work early, which meant they would have to make substantial investments before knowing the results of the trial. It was a major financial risk, and one that manufacturers were reluctant to take. After all, if the results were negative, if the vaccine was not effective, their investment would have been money down the drain. The Foundation dealt with that by guaranteeing the purchase of $9 million worth of vaccine in advance, whatever the outcome of the trial.

In April 1955 Francis delivered his report amid a frenzy of media interest. The vaccine was judged to be 60–70 per cent effective against type I and over 90 per cent effective against II and III. The news leaked out before Francis had finished speaking. 'Diphtheria and tuberculosis had killed many more thousands of children than had polio, but church bells had not greeted the control of these diseases.'[2] The difference may have been due to the work that the Foundation's public relations department had done. Just two hours later the Secretary of Health Education and Welfare had approved licensing the vaccine.

Immediately, discussion of the desirability of polio vaccination began in many countries. In Denmark, which had been shaken by an epidemic of unprecedented severity in 1952, action was rapid. Experts from the Danish Serum Institute had already been in touch with Salk and the Institute quickly set about vaccine production. Other European countries moved more cautiously. In the

Netherlands a specially established committee of the Dutch Health Council (*Gezondheidsraad*) was not convinced that an inactivated vaccine would be effective enough. The minister of health was advised not to permit import of the vaccine. But then, in 1956, the country experienced a serious polio epidemic, to which some two thousand people succumbed. That fact, combined with the clear evidence of what had been achieved in the USA, led to a change of heart. In December 1956 the Netherlands began to import polio vaccine being produced in Belgium, and in 1959 the RIV began work on its own inactivated vaccine.

Meanwhile, some producers were having problems with the production process. Some batches of vaccine had to be discarded because live virus was found in them. It soon became known that six children in California had become paralysed as a result, it was concluded, of vaccine produced by one of the American manufacturers, the Cutter Company. Faced with an agonizing decision – whether to take the Cutter vaccine off the market or suspend the whole programme (after all, everyone was having problems and the disaster could easily recur) – the surgeon general of the USA decided on the former course of action. The Cutter Company stopped production and withdrew supplies of its vaccine. Scientists began to debate whether complete inactivation using formalin (the procedure used) was possible. Perhaps it would be better to inactivate using ultraviolet radiation? In May 1955 the U.S. vaccination programme was briefly suspended. Public faith in the Salk vaccine had been severely shaken.

Most virologists, who were anyway sceptical of the value of an inactivated vaccine, felt vindicated. A number of them were engaged in developing an alternative vaccine, a live attenuated-virus vaccine. These included Hilary Koprowski (a Polish emigré who had worked on a yellow fever vaccine in Brazil) and the very experienced Herald Cox. Both Koprowski and Cox were employed by the pharmaceutical company Lederle where they were both, independently of each other, trying to develop a live-virus vaccine. Lederle had actually begun to work on a live polio vaccine before the existence of three types was known, and had been involved in a premature test on a group of 'mentally defective' children. By modern standards both irresponsible and unethical, this work nevertheless led to an important discovery. Excreted virus was found in their faeces. This implied that as it found its way into the water supply it could protect unvaccinated children in the 'natural' way. This argument was soon to become important when the relative benefits of the different vaccines were being weighed up. On the other hand there was a risk that this excreted attenuated virus might revert to virulence. Both Cox and Koprowski wanted to organize large-scale trials of their vaccines, but there was a problem. Because so many American children had been given Salk vaccine they already had polio antibodies. It would be impossible to distinguish the effects of any new vaccine from those of the older one. The trials would have to be done elsewhere. Finally Koprowski was able to arrange a trial of a two-type vaccine in Northern Ireland, and this started in 1956. Volunteers did not get polio, and they had increased antibodies. However, large amounts of virus were found to be excreted, and much of it had indeed become virulent in its passage through the children's intestines. George Dick, the Belfast professor of microbiology who had arranged the trial, reported negatively. The vaccine was not safe and should not be used on a large scale. Koprowski subsequently left Lederle for the Wistar Institute in Philadelphia and carried out further trials of his polio vaccine in central Africa. Cox remained, continuing his work in Latin America with the support of the Pan American Health Organization.

At the University of Cincinnati Albert Sabin was also working on attenuated polio vaccine, with support from the Foundation. Sabin, who had been born in what was then Russia and emigrated with his parents as a teenager, was able to arrange that his vaccine be tested in the USSR as well as in Poland and Czechoslovakia. In 1957 he sent samples of his three strains to Smorodintsev and Chumakov in the USSR, who would organize its distribution. The preparation was suspended in syrup or candy and then administered to millions of people: more a large-scale demonstration project than a clinical trial. Still, by 1959 positive results were coming in from Eastern Europe. In the United States Joseph Melnick, a professor of virology and epidemiology at Baylor University, was asked to review data relating to the Cox and Sabin vaccines. Melnick wasn't totally happy with either, but much less happy with Cox's, which he decided was too virulent. In August 1960, and despite opposition from the March of Dimes, which felt that the long-term benefits of the Salk vaccine hadn't yet been established, the surgeon general announced that he would recommend licensing the Sabin vaccine. This happened on a strain-by-strain basis, starting with type I in August 1961 and ending with type III (which appeared the most problematic) only in March 1962. At this point Lederle abandoned its own efforts and contracted to manufacture the Sabin vaccine. Vaccines against the three types (I, II and III) were administered separately until a trivalent vaccine, containing all three, was produced in 1963.

The stage was now set for a controversy regarding the relative merits of Salk's inactivated polio vaccine (generally known as IPV) and Sabin's attenuated vaccine. Most virologists thought that the live attenuated vaccine would be better. Since it was administered orally rather than injected, it should be more acceptable to the public. Second, the repeated booster jabs said to be needed with Salk's vaccine would not be necessary since the Sabin vaccine, generally known as the oral polio vaccine, or OPV, was believed to confer longer-lasting immunity. Third, it was quicker acting, immunity being achieved in a matter of days rather than months, which meant that it could be used in the event of a local epidemic. And finally there was the argument that OPV could provide protection to a whole community, and therefore offer a route to ultimate eradication of the virus, thanks to indirect protection resulting from attenuated live virus, excreted into the sewage system. In the 1960s, in parallel with growing medical preference for OPV, pharmaceutical companies in the United States abandoned production of the Salk vaccine. While in the mid-1960s some four to five million doses of IPV were being distributed annually in the USA, by 1967 this had fallen to 2.7 million, and a year later to zero. By contrast, distribution of OPV had reached some 25 million doses annually.

In the summer of 1962, with millions of doses of oral vaccine having been swallowed by American children, a cloud appeared on the horizon. There was a hint that in a small number of cases the attenuated virus in the vaccine had become virulent and itself infected the child with polio. Careful analysis of national data suggested that sixteen cases of polio were probably due to the vaccine itself. While some now recommended that the live-vaccine programme be suspended, others were worried at possible repercussions. What if public faith in the vaccine were so severely shaken that vaccination levels plummeted? Two years later a new committee of enquiry once more reviewed the data. Of the 87 cases of paralytic polio reported since 1961, 57 were judged 'compatible' with having been caused by the OPV itself. This time there was no association with specific lots of vaccine or particular manufacturers. What to do?[3]

Matters were quite different in the Netherlands and the Nordic countries, where IPV produced by the countries' public health institutes was being used very effectively (as it also was in parts of Canada). Under the leadership of Hans Cohen, the Dutch State Institute of Public Health, RIV, had combined inactivated polio vaccine with the DPT that was the mainstay of the country's immunization programme. The idea of combining antigens was not new. Despite worries that antigens could interfere with each other, the first attempts at producing combination vaccines had been made decades earlier. The justification has always been that fewer injections would be needed. In the Netherlands the new combination DPT-P vaccine was used to great effect and polio was brought under control. Subsequently, and despite the absence of an export market (since virtually the whole world was using oral vaccine) the Institute invested considerable resources both in enhancing the potency of the vaccine and in making the production process less dependent on a large supply of monkeys. The Institute was not interested in market opportunities. Innovation had been directed by the needs of the country's highly effective immunization programme. Later the Institute collaborated with Jonas Salk and Charles Mérieux (who were interested both in commercial opportunity and in reinstating IPV) in conducting African trials of the 'enhanced' IPV. The oral vaccine wasn't stable in tropical conditions and required a complex 'cold chain' from site of production to site of delivery. While IPV had the advantage of being far more stable in a hot climate, it would be necessary to convince a sceptical world that it was sufficiently effective in hot countries.

A Golden Age

The attempts to develop new vaccines against viral diseases that followed Enders's work of the 1940s were not limited to polio. Enders's research on viruses had actually started with the mumps virus. Research on the polio virus was initially a sideline for him, albeit one that must soon have come to be seen as the more important, given the widespread fear of polio epidemics. In the developing world polio didn't inspire the same dread. For the poor nations of Africa, Asia and Latin America it was another line of Enders's work at Harvard that would prove of far greater public health importance.

Catching measles, in the 1950s, was something that most North American or West European children went through. It was unpleasant, and it generally meant being confined to a darkened room for some days, but it was rarely serious. Almost all children recovered without any serious consequences. But for an African child catching measles was very serious (as it still is). There, far more children died from measles than from polio. Later there would be more insight into why measles was so much more serious in Africa than in Europe. Many children in poor countries suffer from malnutrition, and this is now understood to compromise the working of their immune systems. But it was also to do with the availability of resources and the new antibiotics. Measles-related deaths were largely due to secondary infections and in the industrialized world these could be treated effectively with antibiotics. Though deaths from measles were falling, incidence of the disease was not, and because the disease was so widespread, absolute numbers were significant and the burden on physicians considerable. Parents did not seem to regard measles as terribly serious, and there was little public pressure for a vaccine. On the other hand the general view among doctors in the United States was that if there were a vaccine, vaccination against measles would be desirable.

John Enders was among those interested in developing a measles vaccine (in contrast to his earlier lack of interest in a polio vaccine). Building on his earlier success with the polio virus, in 1954 Enders and his Harvard colleagues succeeded in culturing the measles virus. Because their initial sample was taken from a boy named David Edmonston, the strain became known as the Edmonston strain. By 1960, together with paediatrician Samuel Katz, Enders had shown that the Edmonston strain, suitably attenuated, stimulated production of measles antibodies in susceptible children. In the spirit of that time, Enders (like Salk) had no interest in patenting his discoveries. On the contrary, because he wanted to encourage other investigators, Enders made the strain freely available to any researcher who wanted to work on it. Very soon many were, including Anton Schwarz at American Home Products and Maurice

Hilleman at Merck. In addition, inspired by Salk's earlier development of an inactivated polio vaccine, other laboratories were trying to develop an inactivated (killed-virus) vaccine.

In March 1963 the first two commercial measles vaccines were approved for use in the United States: a live attenuated vaccine produced by Merck (named Rubeovax) and a formalin-inactivated one produced by Pfizer (known as Pfizer-Vax Measles-K). The live attenuated vaccine appeared to offer children long-term protection against measles. There were nasty side effects though. Many children developed temporary high fevers and a rash after vaccination. Though the side effects could be reduced by giving them gamma globulin (a protein made from blood plasma) at the same time, it was clear that the virus in the vaccine would have to be further attenuated. Inactivated vaccine did not produce these side effects, but based on measurement of antibody levels it also seemed to be less effective. It was unclear whether inactivated-virus vaccine could provide more than a few months' protection. If protection was of too short duration, there was a risk of measles infection being postponed to an older age, when its effects were potentially more serious. A combined schedule was also tried. If a dose of inactivated vaccine was given a month or so before the live vaccine, it seemed that side effects produced by the live vaccine were greatly reduced.

In the U.S. there was rapid political commitment to use of the measles vaccine: indeed within a short time a campaign to eliminate measles from the country had been launched. In Britain, by contrast, even the medical profession was not immediately convinced that the country should embark on mass vaccination against measles. Even if it were to be introduced, it was far from clear which vaccine was to be used, or at what age children should be vaccinated. Starting in 1964, the Medical Research Council set up a trial. In one arm of the trial children were given a live attenuated vaccine (either that produced by Glaxo or by Wellcome), while in the other arm they were first given Pfizer's killed vaccine followed by one of the live vaccines. The single-dose groups seemed to do better, as measured by antibody levels. But then reports from the U.S. began to appear of a strange measles-like illness ('atypical measles') in children given the killed vaccine. An almost universal preference for the live vaccine emerged, and in the U.S. the killed-virus vaccine was withdrawn from the market. In Britain, although no case of 'atypical measles' had been found, when mass measles vaccination began, in 1968, it was with domestically produced live vaccine alone.

In principle a killed vaccine ought to be safer, though there was no evidence that a live measles vaccine could revert to virulence. But experience with the polio vaccines, when in a very few cases polio was caused by the virus in the vaccine becoming virulent, was fresh in people's memories. Some virologists thought that the idea of a killed measles virus vaccine had been written off prematurely. Erling Norrby, professor at the Karolinska Institute in Stockholm, had been working on a measles vaccine since 1959. He was convinced that the strange effects the killed vaccine seemed to produce could be avoided if the virus was inactivated in a different way. Instead of formalin, an organic solvent known as Tween-ether was used, and it seemed that this would destroy the agents that produced the strange reactions that had been seen in the u.s. The Dutch too, thinking back to their success with polio, preferred an inactivated vaccine. In the hope of replicating the strategy that had been so successful earlier, they wanted to combine an inactivated measles vaccine with the quadrivalent vaccine (DPT-P) already in use. At both Glaxo and Behringwerke studies of inactivated measles vaccine were also going on, and to start with, Dutch researchers discussed the possibility of obtaining a measles strain from them. In the end, however, they turned to Norrby in Sweden. With a strain obtained from Sweden they produced a DTP/polio/inactivated measles vaccine, which in 1971 was tested in clinical trials in the Netherlands. Unfortunately, however, the protection it provided proved to decline so rapidly that the vaccine would not be of any use. The decision was taken to terminate the work and to purchase a strain from Merck.

Scientists were also working on vaccines against rubella (also known as German measles). Before 1940 this had not been considered a particularly serious disease. However, in 1940 Norman Gregg, an Australian ophthalmologist, found a link between a rubella infection in pregnancy and the birth of a baby with defective vision. It was subsequently established that if it was contracted during pregnancy rubella could lead to spontaneous abortion, to central nervous system defects, or to one of a range of other serious and debilitating conditions in a newborn child (known as 'congenital rubella syndrome'). In the mid-1960s the USA was struck by a

particularly serious rubella epidemic, and public pressure to produce a vaccine built up. Again, many laboratories set about it, using
different strains and different attenuation processes. Most of them
were culturing the virus on monkey or rabbit kidney cells. Somewhat
controversially, at the Wistar Institute in Philadelphia, Stanley
Plotkin grew his virus in a culture made from aborted foetuses.
Though many objected on moral grounds, or disagreed on technical
grounds, Plotkin felt that this would ensure they were free of the
contaminating pathogens found in many animal cell cultures. The
vaccine that he developed was called RA27/3, and by the end of the
1960s it had been adopted by a number of European manufacturers (including Burroughs Wellcome in the UK and Institut Mérieux
in France), though American companies were hesitant. By 1970 a
number of rubella vaccines were being produced, both commercially
and (in the Netherlands) in the public sector.

Given the known extent of foetal death and malformation it
caused, medical professionals agreed on the value of a vaccine
against rubella. But evaluating the different rubella vaccines, and
deciding which to use, was particularly protracted and complex.
Control of rubella presented a unique problem because the ultimate
goal was protection of a foetus against damage from intrauterine
infection before it had even been conceived. The possibility of
immunity declining with time, so that women would have reduced
immunity by the time they reached childbearing age, then became
particularly vital. Despite studies showing little difference between
the vaccines, or complex and varying changes in immunity over
time, consensus in favour of the RA27/3 vaccines emerged, on the
grounds that they appeared to provide longer-lasting immunity. In
1978 the decision was taken at Merck to replace the strain they had
been using with the RA27/3 strain, and this was finally licensed in
the United States in January 1979.

Today most people in the industrialized world encounter measles and rubella vaccines as two components of a three-component
vaccine known as MMR. Despite questions having recently been asked
regarding possible adverse effects (which we will discuss later),
this combination vaccine is one of the foundations of vaccination
programmes in most industrialized countries. What of the third
component: mumps? Though it was his success with the polio virus
that brought him fame, John Enders's research on viral diseases

had actually begun with mumps. The most familiar symptom of mumps is a swelling of the salivary glands below the ear called the parotid glands, though many people who catch mumps develop no symptoms at all. In a few cases complications were known to arise, notably aseptic meningitis (or mumps encephalitis), but these were rare, and as antibiotics became available they could be treated successfully. Widespread popular belief notwithstanding, male sterility very rarely followed mumps infection. After initially failing to grow the virus in cell culture, Enders and Joseph Stokes had produced a vaccine by making an emulsion from infected parotid monkey glands and inactivating it with formalin. It was tried out first in monkeys and then in human volunteers. In 1948 Enders's laboratory managed to grow the virus in tissue culture made from fragments of chick embryo and were then able to produce an attenuated virus vaccine by numerous passages through embryonated eggs. In the USSR, Smorodintsev in Leningrad was working along similar lines.

Was a mumps vaccine needed? Vaccines developed up to this time had rarely provoked major doubts as to their value in professional circles. Nevertheless, the widely held view among European medical professionals was that, though unpleasant, childhood mumps was a mild disease. Though physicians in the u.s. may have thought differently, in the 1960s and '70s their British and European colleagues were not convinced that a mumps vaccine was needed. In the Netherlands, the Institute of Public Health, though very active in the fields of polio and measles vaccine development, didn't consider trying to develop a mumps vaccine because they didn't think it would be required.

Others clearly thought differently, and were trying to develop mumps vaccines using virus strains circulating locally. Because laboratories started with different strains and used different attenuation procedures, big differences between the vaccines emerged. The first mumps vaccines appeared in 1967. The Leningrad-3 strain was produced by the Leningrad Influenza Institute using cultures made from guinea pig kidney cells, and subsequently further attenuated by passages through Japanese quail embryo cultures. This vaccine was produced and used in the former Soviet Union and elsewhere, and continues to be widely used internationally. In the same year, Merck's Mumpsvax was licensed in the USA. Under the leadership of Maurice Hilleman, Merck had started work on a live attenuated mumps vaccine in 1959, apparently with the goal of including it as part of a multi-component vaccine. A virus strain was taken from Hilleman's daughter and was named 'Jeryl Lynn' after her. Trials had shown that the vaccine was safe and effective in a single dose: there seemed to be no side effects and immunity persisted at least for a number of months. Many other mumps vaccines followed, of which widely used ones include the Urabe strain, developed in Japan, and the L-Zagreb. This was produced at the Institute of Immunology in Zagreb (in what is now Croatia) by further attenuating the Leningrad-3 strain. L-Zagreb has also been widely used internationally.

To what extent did development of these mumps vaccines reflect the burden of the disease? Was it a matter of widely differ- ent assessments of the health risk posed by mumps? Or was there a sense that anything that could be prevented should be prevented?

In just a few years, the combined MMR vaccine would make this question redundant. Combinations of antigens have to be tested in extensive trials, just like wholly new antigens. The various com- ponents might interfere with one another, and any deleterious consequences must be ruled out. The diphtheria-pertussis-tetanus vaccine (DPT) had been in use for some years, so it was clear that combining antigens was in principle feasible. Dutch researchers had gone on successfully to combine the Salk polio vaccine with the DPT in order to keep down the number of separate visits to the child health centre that would be needed. Merck did not produce DPT, so they were interested in other possible combinations. Recognizing that there could be a number of advantages in combining anti- gens, Maurice Hilleman, who ran Merck's vaccine development programme, had begun studying antibody responses to various com- binations in the late 1960s. Among the combinations he tried out was a three-component measles, mumps and rubella vaccine. This is what Merck decided to produce and MMR vaccine was licensed in the USA in 1971, alongside the individual vaccines. While compet- ing manufacturers produced the individual vaccines, Merck soon became the country's only domestic supplier of MMR vaccine. From a public health point of view the major argument for combining different antigens was, and is, that schedules can be simplified, and uptake thus increased. Clearly the greater the problem of achiev- ing high coverage rates, the greater the benefit from a combined multiantigen vaccine. Since low coverage rates had long been a matter of concern in the USA the combination vaccine had particular advantages there, and MMR began to be used routinely by the mid-1970s. The commercial benefits to Merck are obvious. In Western Europe coverage rates were higher, and introduction of the combined MMR vaccine took place later, and for slightly different reasons.

The Vaccine Industry at Mid-century

Producing the new viral vaccines had presented both scientists and manufacturers with a host of new challenges. Methods that had been developed for producing the previous generation of bacterial vaccines had had to be radically adapted. Some, such as the influenza virus, could be grown in hen's eggs. In other cases, notably the polio virus, finding a suitable medium in which it could be safely cultured required a major breakthrough. From an organizational point of view, however, relatively little changed between the 1920s and the 1960s. Initial research and development would often be carried out in a university or government laboratory, or by some kind of collaboration, and production would then take place in different kinds of institution. Vaccine development and production in the middle decades of the twentieth century was still shared between public- and private-sector institutions, often in easy collaboration. Thus polio and measles vaccines, like the older vaccines already in widespread use (DPT, smallpox, BCG), were produced by a wide variety of institutions. Some were long-established pharmaceutical companies, bearing the names of their founders well into the 1960s or '70s: Eli Lilly in the U.S., Behringwerke in (West) Germany, Burroughs Wellcome in the UK, Connaught in Canada, Institut Mérieux in France, Sclavo in Italy. There were a few newcomers. For example, in Belgium Recherche et Industrie Thérapeutique (RIT), founded in the 1940s, was an early producer of the Salk polio vaccine.

While in Britain, Germany and the United States vaccines were supplied almost exclusively by commercial producers like these, this was not the case everywhere. In the communist states of Central and Eastern Europe vaccine supply was the responsibility of the state. In the Dutch and Scandinavian welfare states too, producing the vaccines that public health services required was seen as part of the state's responsibility. In parts of Africa and Asia, institutes of public health that had been established years previously by colonial administrations, or by the Pasteur Institute or the Rockefeller Foundation, were taken over by the governments of newly independent states. Political movements focused on industrialization could also influence developments, as for example in Mexico, where the Instituto Nacional de Virología was proud of its ability to produce all the paediatric vaccines the country needed. There were many countries in which both public-sector and private manufacturers contributed – countries as different in their political histories as Australia, Brazil, China, India, South Africa and Turkey.

In the 1950s and '60s there was no deep ideological divide between vaccine scientists working in the East and the West, whatever the Cold War rhetoric. Nor, in the West, was there any deep ideological divide between public- and private-sector manufacturers. Certainly in Europe, their relationships were typically rooted in a common commitment to public health, whether or not allied to a need to make a profit. Knowledge was freely available and freely exchanged. Patents played little or no role in vaccine development at this time, and flows of virus strains or know-how were scarcely hindered by commercial interests. Jonas Salk, who donated his virus strains to the who and assigned all patent rights to the organization, thought patenting in this field immoral. As he famously remarked: 'Can you patent the sun?' Hans Cohen, who was for many years director general of the Netherlands State Institute (RIVM) responsible for producing and supplying the country's vaccines, tells of his earlier relationships with industry, specifically with Pasteur Mérieux (now part of Sanofi-Aventis):

> They [Mérieux] got all our know-how, and we weren't always happy about that, but on the other hand we got a great deal of know-how back in return. For example, I got a rabies vaccine. We exchanged. It took three minutes. A matter of 'what do you want from me?' then the boss says 'I'll have some polio, and what do you want?' And I'd say 'Give me a measles strain, and some of that and some of that . . .' It was good. Really a free exchange.[4]

State vaccine institutions were at the mercy of political shifts, and in some parts of the world (though less so in Europe) this could significantly affect their budgets and stability. On the other hand they were more or less immune to market forces – which of course was not true of commercial manufacturers. As vaccines appeared to be gaining or losing their commercial promise, companies began or abandoned vaccine production and the industry grew or shrunk. In the 1960s the commercial promise of the new viral vaccines brought new players to the industry. In Europe, for example, SmithKline French acquired RIT in 1963, in order to enter the vaccine market. In 1968, Rhône-Poulenc took over the Institut Mérieux, founded in 1897 by an assistant to Pasteur. In the United States the number of licensed manufacturers grew in response to both the new scientific possibilities, and the more active role being taken by the federal government in promoting vaccination. Industrial commitment, however, was to prove uncertain and unreliable.

If and when the vaccine market became less attractive, a company could always devote itself wholly to the production of pharmaceuticals. In the USA this is precisely what happened in the 1970s. From the mid-1960s to the end of the 1970s the number of licensed vaccine manufacturers fell by half, and even the number of licensed vaccine products fell. Like the majority of Western industrialized countries, the United States was almost wholly dependent on private pharmaceutical companies for its supplies of vaccines. ('Almost' because the departments of public health of the states of Massachusetts and Michigan had facilities that produced some vaccines for the inhabitants of their states.) As far as nineteen vaccines, including the polio vaccine, were concerned, there was only a single American producer. What if that producer decided to stop making vaccines? There were precedents enough. For example, in the mid-1970s, Eli Lilly was working on an experimental pneumococcal vaccine with support from the National Institutes of Health (NIH). Then, for commercial reasons, the company decided to terminate almost all its vaccine research and development and production activities. The vulnerability of the vaccine supply system was becoming a matter of political concern in the USA. The Congressional Office of Technology Assessment (OTA), investigating the matter, felt that 'the apparently diminishing commitment – and possibly capacity – of the American pharmaceutical industry to research, develop, and produce vaccines ... may be reaching levels of real concern.'[5] Company executives told the OTA that this reflected the costs and difficulties of developing vaccines, market considerations and carrying out the testing of each batch of vaccine as required by federal regulations. Regulatory oversight had been strengthened. Vaccines were more difficult to develop, test and license than pharmaceutical products. They were also less profitable, and there were much greater risks of liability actions and huge damages if anything went wrong. And when they did, as indeed they did, the federal government had to step in to ensure the industry – and so the nation's vaccine supply – remained viable.

From a global perspective this is not the whole story, however. In 1966 the World Health Organization committed itself seriously to the global eradication of smallpox. This globally coordinated smallpox vaccination campaign (about which more later) would make use of a thermally stable freeze-dried vaccine that was being produced in the Soviet Union. The scale of the operation was so great that local vaccine producers in smallpox-endemic countries would also have to contribute if the supply was going to be adequate. But international experts were dubious as to the quality of much that they produced. It would be important to ensure that their products were of adequate quality. So not only would local production have to be stimulated through technology transfer, but the international system of quality control would have to be strengthened as well. So, in parallel with changes starting to take place in the North American and European vaccine industries, the WHO was assisting developing-country manufacturers improve the scale and quality of their vaccine production. These efforts bore fruit, so that local producers in India, Iran, Kenya and several Latin American countries were able to donate smallpox vaccine to neighbouring countries. Later, it was estimated that developing-country manufacturers produced at least 80 per cent of the vaccine needed in the developing world.

Well into the 1970s, the WHO remained committed to encouraging and extending local or regional vaccine production and supply, and to the transfer of technology to local producers. Only a few institutes in developing countries (notably in Brazil, Mexico and India) had the capacity to produce the newer vaccines such as those against polio and measles. Nevertheless in many countries of the developing world, meeting the country's vaccine needs – vaccine self-sufficiency – fitted well with 1960s political rhetoric and with the political aspirations of national leaders.

FOUR

TECHNOLOGIES: THE COMMODIFICATION OF VACCINES

Changing Priorities

The vaccines developed in the first six or seven decades of the twentieth century have saved literally countless lives. Though the fit certainly was not perfect, vaccine development tended to be in response to healthcare need. The fit was not perfect, principally in the sense that the healthcare needs that inspired vaccine development were largely those of the industrialized world. There was little interest in developing vaccines needed only in very poor countries, since those countries would not have the resources with which to purchase them. For example, despite the fact that parasitic diseases were responsible for a great deal of sickness and death in tropical countries, there were no vaccines and little effort was devoted to developing them. Of course, some of the vaccines developed in response to health concerns of the industrialized countries, especially those against whooping cough and measles, had benefited everybody. But what now of the more recent period, from the 1980s onwards? To what extent has healthcare need continued to 'drive' vaccine development? And in so far as it has, whose healthcare need? And if it has not, what has taken its place? Many new vaccines have become available in the last twenty to thirty years. Is this because human beings now face challenges from a growing number of infectious pathogens? And if not, then what explains the stream of new vaccines?

The context in which public health policy was formulated, and in which vaccine development took place, was transformed in the 1980s. The most visible and dramatic change was, of course, the fall of the Berlin wall and the collapse of the Soviet Union at the decade's end. But prior to that, other changes had been taking place.

An economic crisis had devastating and widespread consequences. Some economies, such as that of Argentina, crashed. Across the developing world wages were falling, poverty and unemployment were rising and governments were unable to pay their bills. It was at this time that, under the influence of the U.S. Treasury and State Department, international aid organizations adopted an extreme ideological commitment to liberalization, deregulation and privatization. The implications of this ideological shift for the organization and provision of healthcare were profound and immediate and we will come back to them later. So far as vaccine development is concerned the consequences, though less direct, were nevertheless significant. It is on these consequences that we focus in this chapter.

In 1984 the influential U.S. Institute of Medicine (IOM) began an investigation intended to identify the vaccines most needed in developing countries and which, on the basis of existing knowledge, it ought to be possible to produce within a decade. The rotavirus had been isolated some years earlier. The respiratory syncytial virus (RSV), which can cause pneumonia and is especially risky for children with compromised immune systems such as premature babies, had been identified in 1956. A formalin-inactivated RSV vaccine had actually been made in the 1960s, but had been withdrawn because the protection it offered was too short-lived. *Streptococcus pneumoniae* bacteria ('pneumococcus'), which can cause many types of illnesses, including pneumonia, ear infections, sinus infections, meningitis (infection of the covering around the brain and spinal cord) and bacteremia (bloodstream infection), had actually been isolated by Louis Pasteur. Malaria was more complicated, even though its cause – certain species of a parasite known as plasmodium – had also been identified in the previous century. A 1950s campaign to eradicate malaria through attacking the mosquito that carries the parasite, with swamp drainage, bed nets and chemicals, had failed. There had been attempts at developing a malaria vaccine since the 1940s, though all had failed. What made development of a malaria vaccine so difficult was the parasite's complex life cycle.

Looking at potential health benefits as well as the state of play, the IOM listed the vaccines that were not only needed but seemingly within reach.[1] Vaccines against *S. pneumoniae*, malaria, rotavirus and shigella figured prominently on their list, while other diseases, including hepatitis B and RSV became priorities under certain assumptions. The IOM committee found that few of their priority vaccines had attracted any interest from the pharmaceutical industry. If these vaccines were to be developed, the IOM argued, the Federal government would have to step in. A decade later, a survey carried out by the journal *Science* found that there was still no vaccine against any of the diseases that had been given highest priority by the IOM.[2] Two of the vaccines that figured lower down the list had been developed. Significantly, these two, against haemophilus influenza (HiB) and against hepatitis B (HepB), also had important markets in the industrialized world, and what is more had been priced far out of the reach of poor countries.

Lack of industrial interest in the vaccines that poor countries most needed was a major concern for researchers who wondered whether their work would ever be turned into life-saving innovations. The *Science* article quotes from an interview with a prominent parasitologist, Ruth Nussenzweig, who explains that in the 1980s it had been impossible to interest any pharmaceutical company: 'They'd turn their back when the word "malaria" was announced.'[3] Nussenzweig went on to criticize the lack of coordination in the field and the fact that the U.S. government, especially the U.S. Agency for International Development (USAID), which had once invested substantially in malaria research, had reduced its commitment. Vaccines against malaria, pneumococcus and rotavirus would undoubtedly offer enormous social benefit, but companies doubted that they'd get much of a return on investments of the tens of millions of dollars it cost to develop a new vaccine. The rich countries of the industrial north were hardly likely to embark on large-scale malaria vaccination, and poor countries would not be able to afford the vaccine when it had been developed. Not that lack of interest in vaccines against parasitic diseases was anything new. But in the 1980s public health priorities on the one hand and investment decisions on the other seemed to be moving further and further apart. What had happened? After all, not so long before it had not been like that. Vaccine development had more or less corresponded to health need. At the institutional level there were public-sector vaccine institutes, like the Dutch RIVM, whose research and development work directly reflected the needs of the national immunization programme, and which was committed to transferring vaccine technology to poor countries. But by the early years of the new millennium almost no such institutes remained in the industrialized world, and links between health priorities and investment in vaccine development had been fractured. Noting the changes taking place in the late 1980s, two knowledgeable insiders wrote:

> Public health objectives and advocacy . . . do not drive business decisions, and vaccine development often stalls when commercial firms calculate the relative advantage of investing in vaccines versus other products. Ultimately, industry executives, not public health officials, make the decisions about which products to develop.[4]

Developments in political economy on the one hand and science and technology on the other were bringing about a fundamental change both in priority-setting and in the way vaccines were developed. New techniques for manipulating genetic material promised entirely new ways of producing vaccines precision-tailored to do a very specific job. The scientists who had mastered these new techniques worked in universities or in non-profit research institutes and centres, not in the pharmaceutical industry. Traditional vaccine manufacturers, whether multinational pharmaceutical companies or national institutes of public health, lacked expertise in techniques of genetic manipulation. In 1980 the u.s. Congress passed legislation, the Bayh–Dole Act, pushing universities to license patentable research done with government funding to private corporations, instead of requiring them to grant the patents to the federal government. Significant numbers of scientists who had been working on the manipulation of genetic material moved out of the university into small, high-tech 'spin-off' firms. It was here that the expertise that the larger vaccine manufacturers would soon covet was to be found. Producing nothing to begin with, their expertise was these companies' sole resource. As the treasure they would exhibit in order to raise capital on the stock market, it had to be jealously guarded through patenting as extensively as possible.

Internationally, too, the knowledge on which companies like these – as well as the giant pharmaceutical companies – depended was acquiring a new and more highly protected status. Prior to the mid-1990s, there were major international differences in countries' patent laws. In some countries patenting of medicines was not permitted, on the grounds that they were vital for people's health. At the talks on international trade taking place in the early 1990s (the so-called Uruguay Round of talks on reduction of tariffs) the decision was taken to establish a new organization to be known as the World Trade Organization (WTO). At the urging of the U.S. delegation, supported by its European and Japanese counterparts, membership of the new organization, which would carry with it numerous benefits in the area of international trade, was made conditional on modifications to national patent laws. In 1995, at the end of years of negotiation, the agreement known as TRIPS, or Trade-related Aspects of Intellectual Property Rights, came into force. The restrictions it placed on, for example, the production of generic anti-retroviral medicines led to protests mounted by developing countries supported by a number of campaigning NGOs. A few years later the so-called Doha Declaration clarified the grounds on which it was permissible to circumvent TRIPS provisions, for example in the event of a public health emergency. Multinational pharmaceutical companies, unhappy with this revision, which they viewed as damaging to their interests, sought additional forms of protection. The result of their lobbying has been a set of largely bilateral agreements between the governments of industrialized countries (notably the United States) and developing countries, which contain additional and more stringent provisions. All of this has become known as 'TRIPS plus'. A great deal has been written about the treaties, the protests, the revisions and the implications for the availability of locally manufactured generic medicines. The crucial point here is simply this. The knowledge on which the production of new vaccines would be based was being 'privatized', turned into private 'intellectual property'. Justified on the grounds that developing valuable drugs and vaccines cost a great deal of money, the new arrangements were intended to keep 'intellectual property' well guarded, locally and internationally.

How did it all work in practice? The first vaccine to be developed using the new techniques, and under this new intellectual-property regime, offered protection against hepatitis B – to those who could afford it.

New Tools and a New Context: Hepatitis B

Hepatitis is an infection of the liver, with symptoms that have been known since ancient times. It may go away by itself or it may lead to cirrhosis or cancer of the liver many years later. In the nineteenth century doctors began to suspect that there might be more than one kind of hepatitis. What until the 1960s was generally called 'infectious hepatitis', now known as hepatitis A, is spread by the faecal/oral route. The virus is spread, for example, when an infected person fails to clean his or her hands thoroughly after use of the toilet and then handles food. Hepatitis A is the most common type and, though highly contagious, rarely has serious long-term effects. Another hepatitis, with what looked like similar symptoms, seemed to be associated with blood and was clearly transmitted in a different way. This 'other' hepatitis (B) became known as 'serum hepatitis', because it appeared in populations receiving blood transfusions, or having come into contact with contaminated needles or blood. (Hepatitis C was characterized in 1989 and another four forms thereafter. But hepatitis A and B are the most common.) The difference between hepatitis A and B was understood largely as a result of studies that had involved the deliberate infection of institutionalized children with intellectual disabilities. It would later be established that hepatitis B is not only spread through blood, but also through sexual contact, from mother to baby, and even through casual contact in households. In 1964 an almost fortuitous discovery by the American geneticist Baruch Blumberg led to a breakthrough in the understanding of hepatitis. Investigating differential susceptibility to various diseases, using blood samples from around the world, Blumberg found an intriguing protein in the blood of an Australian aboriginal. Subsequent work by Blumberg and by Alfred Prince at the New York Blood Center showed that this was an antigen (a surface protein) of the hepatitis B virus. Somewhat later, D. S. Dane at London's Middlesex Hospital identified the complete virus, which turned out to be quite different from any other known virus family. Thanks to these discoveries it became possible to test serologically for the presence of this antigen, and so for the first time to see if someone had hepatitis B, or if a blood supply was contaminated with the virus. Blumberg received a 1976 Nobel Prize for this work. No one could have anticipated that a significant percentage of the world's population carried the hepatitis B virus (though not all developed the disease). Especially in Asia and in southern African countries, 10 or even 20 per cent of the population were carriers. In the United States the carrier rate was far lower, but certain groups were found to be at particular risk of infection. They included recipients of blood transfusions (especially people suffering from haemophilia), healthcare workers who came into contact with blood (such as surgeons, nurses and dentists), sex workers and homosexuals with multiple partners. Hepatitis B was rampant in the gay community in the 1970s. Soldiers stationed in regions such as Southeast Asia, where there was a significant chance that casual sexual partners would be carriers, were also a high-risk group. Hepatitis B attracted little public attention, and when a test became available there were no calls for universal testing, perhaps, historian William Muraskin has suggested, because doctors themselves were a high-risk group.

Blumberg and his colleague Irving Millman went on to develop a hepatitis B vaccine, which was basically a heat-treated form of the virus, and patented it in 1969. Muraskin, who extensively interviewed a number of the leading protagonists, writes that Blumberg expected a large pharmaceutical company to develop the product further. While Merck was interested it insisted on an exclusive licence. When this proved impossible, since NIH had funded Blumberg's work and their rules forbade exclusive licences, Merck withdrew. In the mid-1970s they were, however, given an exclusive licence on markets outside the United States and on that basis proceeded to move ahead.

Because the virus wouldn't grow in cell culture, it was not possible to produce a vaccine in the way that had worked with polio and measles vaccines. Merck's procedure involved harvesting the antigen, now known as HBsAg, from the blood plasma of volunteer carriers. Since this antigen should stimulate the body to produce antibodies to the virus it could be the basis of a vaccine, though it would first have to be purified and very carefully inactivated. The problem would be to get hold of sufficient antigen to start with. Here, a collaboration with Saul Krugman, a professor of paediatrics at New York University School of Medicine who had been studying hepatitis for years, would be crucial. By 1975 Merck had a preparation that they were ready to try on human volunteers. A placebo-controlled trial was then designed in collaboration with the New York Blood Center, to be carried out among the city's gay male population. The results, which came in 1980, were sufficiently positive that in November 1981 Merck's Heptavax-B was approved for sale in the United States. It was put on the market at $100 for the requisite three shots: a price far beyond the reach of many countries in which hepatitis B infection was widespread and need far greater than in the United States. Many people in the public health community were shocked by the price. It had been known that the vaccine would be expensive, because of the fancy technology used in preparing it, but many felt that this price was wholly unjustified.

Blood banks had ready access to plasma and expertise in handling it, and unlike most pharmaceutical companies they were not looking to make as much profit as they could from developing a vaccine. In New York's Blood Center and in the Dutch Blood Transfusion Service Laboratory, work aimed at development of an *affordable* vaccine was also under way.

In New York, Alfred Prince set about perfecting a process that should yield a very much cheaper product (he was thinking of $1 per shot rather than Merck's $33) and – crucially – could be transferred to local manufacturers in countries where it was most needed. Prince was successful, and it seems that his heat inactivation process needed a much smaller amount of the most costly raw material (blood plasma), while producing an equally potent vaccine. Thanks to the mediation of Korean–American contacts in the U.S., a production agreement was reached with the Cheil Sugar Company in Korea, a subsidiary of Samsung. The agreement was warmly supported by James Maynard, chief of the CDC's hepatitis branch, and a leading expert in the field. Maynard shared Prince's commitment to affordable vaccines produced by transferable technology. But problems arose between Prince and Cheil Sugar, as Muraskin has shown.[5] The company moved too hesitantly and lacked a marketing strategy outside Korea. Nor did it have much understanding of the need for well-designed clinical trials that would produce convincing data. When finally the vaccine was ready, the company planned to sell it for $5–8 per dose: much less than Merck, but much more than the $1 that Prince had in mind. However, problems were eventually overcome, and in 1982 the vaccine was put on the market.

In the Netherlands, though the Blood Transfusion Service Laboratory (CLB) had access to plenty of blood plasma, it had no experience of vaccine research. The National Institute of Public Health (RIV) had plenty of the latter, and moreover anticipated that the country would need a hepatitis B vaccine. In the mid-1970s, the two institutions began to collaborate, and with some help from the New York Blood Center, they developed a vaccine that was ready to be tested on human volunteers. At the end of the 1970s a cohort of male homosexual volunteers was set up in Amsterdam. Later, in collaboration with the Thai Red Cross, a trial was carried out in Thailand. The vaccine worked. Though four shots were required, rather than the three recommended with Merck's Heptavax, the end result seemed to be just as good.

These plasma-derived hepatitis B vaccines, as well as others developed by the Korean Green Cross, and by the commercial arm of the Pasteur Institute, were launched in the early 1980s. A couple of years later the HIV/AIDS epidemic broke out in the U.S. Gay men were at particular risk of both hepatitis B and HIV infection, but they quite commonly gave blood too. Might the plasma-derived vaccine be contaminated with HIV virus? A test for presence of the virus only became available in 1985. Before it had been established that the HIV virus was actually killed by the inactivation process, anxiety that the vaccine might be unsafe was spreading. These concerns played an important role in discussions of the safety standards that a vaccine would have to meet. In the event, standards were initially set so high that public-sector institutions like the Korean Green Cross, the Dutch Blood Laboratory and the New York Blood Center were unable to meet them. It is hard to say how far this reflected innate public anxieties, and how far it was due to large pharmaceutical companies putting up hurdles, exaggerating the dangers, so as to drive the smaller players out (as some have suggested).

At the same time, work was starting on a different kind of hepatitis B vaccine, avoiding the use of plasma. A number of arguments were put forward for doing it differently. For example: 'When everyone has been vaccinated there'll be no infected carriers from whom to collect plasma'; or 'It's difficult to collect plasma in some parts of the world.' But safety was the most powerful argument. As Freeman and Robbins wrote in 1991:

> When a Korean manufacturer offered a plasma-derived version at about $1 per dose for a clinical trial organised under

the aegis of the Pan American Health Organization in the Caribbean, makers of the genetically engineered vaccine succeeded in derailing the test by raising unsubstantiated charges that the Korean vaccine was unsafe.[6]

What was this new vaccine? A vaccine consisting of a protein from a virus's outer covering can stimulate an immune reaction but, since it does not contain any genetic material, it carries no risk of becoming virulent. What the new 'genetic engineering' suggested was that such a protein could be produced without starting from infected blood. If the fragment of the viral DNA that coded for the protective protein could be cut out and spliced into a suitable substrate, multiplication of the substrate (for example bacterial cells) would also produce the protein. Attempts to develop innovative products based on these 'recombinant' techniques were in full swing in the early 1980s; not in large pharmaceutical companies like Merck or SmithKline, but in universities and in new biotech companies, such as Genentech, Chiron and Genetic Systems, that had been set up by entrepreneurial scientists and which were patenting aggressively. Both SmithKline and Merck were determined to develop recombinant HepB vaccines, and Merck soon signed a cooperation agreement with Chiron and with two university laboratories. The principle to be applied was that a fragment of DNA coding for the virus's HBsAg surface antigen would be inserted into a yeast cell, where it would cause the yeast to produce the desired antigen in its own replication. By the mid-1980s they had produced the recombinant vaccine. The multistage procedure involved fermenting the yeast and rupturing the yeast cells to release the antigen, which was then separated, purified and inactivated with formaldehyde. Finally, it was adsorbed onto aluminium hydroxide (which served as an adjuvant) and preserved by addition of an organo-mercury compound known as thimerosal. Merck's Recombivax HB, licensed in the USA in 1986, and SmithKline's Engerix B, licensed in Belgium in the same year, were the first vaccines produced by recombinant DNA methods. Business historian Louis Galambos, in his history of Merck's vaccine work, states that SKB offered three doses at $149.20, undercutting Merck's $170.51 (also for three doses).[7] Competition was now taking place on the basis of price as well as effectiveness, though clearly these vaccines were much more expensive than the original Heptavax, let alone the few dollars that the Koreans were charging.

Merck and GSK hepatitis B vaccines are the only ones approved for use in the United States, where the requisite three shots now cost between $75 and $165 for children, and more for adults. But the global market is another matter, since by far the largest hepatitis B burden is found in Asia. In India, where 4 per cent of the population are estimated to be carriers and 100,000 people to die every year from the consequences of a hepatitis B infection, plasma-derived vaccines had been produced since the early 1980s.[8] However, there as elsewhere, concerns arose regarding safety and the sustainability of production. Among the new biotech firms emerging in India, at least one, Shantha Biotechnics, set about trying to develop an affordable recombinant vaccine. In 1997 their domestically produced vaccine, Shanvac-B, was launched at only $1 per dose, with the result that 22 million doses were sold the following year. In 2009 the European multinational Sanofi-Aventis took a controlling share in Shantha.

New Configurations

The ideological shift that took place in the Reagan and Thatcher years, the tidal wave of free-market thinking, had major implications for the development and production of vaccines. The functioning, and the legitimacy, of the public-sector vaccine producers was undermined. Publications emphasized their deficiencies – political interference and inadequate management structures, outdated facilities carrying risks of poor quality vaccines, lack of independent regulation and control – and suggested that their time had passed. Interestingly, the arguments being put forward were pretty much the same as the ones that American pharmaceutical companies had used against the municipal producers of diphtheria serum seventy years before! Many governments, converted to the idea of a minimalist state, concluded that producing vaccines was not something that they should be doing. It was not only that the private sector could do it better or more economically. It was ideological conviction as well as potential economies that led to the closure or privatization of public-sector vaccine institutes, which started in the 1990s in Australia and Sweden. In the United States the state of Michigan, which by this time ran the country's only public-sector vaccine producer, put it up for sale in 1996. There were no bidders for facilities that had been losing millions of dollars and which the *New York Times* called 'rickety'. But this was the country's only licensed producer of anthrax vaccine, and when fears of a bioterrorist attack led to a demand for anthrax vaccine, private-sector interest emerged and the facility was sold in 1998. Ideological as well as economic considerations led to the sale of the Dutch vaccine institute to the Serum Institute of India (a private company) in 2013, of the venerable Danish institute to a Malaysian company in 2016, and to the fact that the government of Croatia is at the time of writing trying to find a purchaser for the Zagreb institute.

The emergence of new ways of making vaccines, and legislation in the United States designed to facilitate the transfer of government-funded research to the private sector, were two factors that catalysed renewed interest in vaccine production on the part of the pharmaceutical industry. There were others. Widespread popular concern at the side effects of the pertussis vaccine had led to a surge in legal actions claiming damages against manufacturers, and in the USA a number of them were considering leaving the vaccine business. In 1986, responding to the political implications of a declining vaccines sector, the U.S. Congress passed legislation establishing a National Childhood Vaccine Injury Compensation Program. This limited the liability of manufacturers and established a public fund from which possible compensation claims could be paid. Suitably reassured, pharmaceutical firms began to reconsider their commitment to vaccines. They courted the young biotech firms that had the skills (and the patents) they lacked, as Merck's recombinant hepatitis B deal with Chiron illustrates. Alongside access to international markets, access to patents has become one of the most important factors in mergers and takeovers in the vaccines field. Pfizer's $68 million takeover of Wyeth Pharmaceuticals in 2009 seems to have been motivated specifically by Pfizer (the world's largest drug company) wishing to re-enter the vaccine field by acquiring Wyeth's patents. (Wyeth had itself taken over Lederle in 1994.)

The costs of testing a new vaccine – of organizing the trials, and of collating the safety and efficacy data required by increasingly stringent regulatory regimes – have been rising constantly, so that today it costs hundreds of millions (of dollars, euros or pounds) to get a new vaccine to the market. In the 1980s it was often pointed out that only the private sector had the necessary resources. Moreover, increasingly focused on maximizing shareholder return on investment, the industry was responding to the new economic climate. Commercial vaccine manufacturers were unwilling to collaborate with those in the public sector as they had done a decade earlier. Scientific knowledge was being privatized and, as a source of potential profit, was now rebranded as 'intellectual property'. Denied access to this new technology, public-sector producers were unable to produce the new vaccines that public health authorities were demanding.

Policy advisers began to argue that ways would have to be found of inducing the commercial pharmaceutical industry to commit itself to developing the vaccines they felt public health systems needed. One suggestion was that partnerships could be set up, linking companies with institutions working in the field of public health, so that there would be a match between what the health sector hoped for and what companies were developing. Relationships that had been taken for granted or as unworthy of comment in the 1970s now became the crux of the issue, providing a key metaphor as well as an institutional structure for today's world: the public–private partnership:

> Public–private partnerships exist at the nexus of several diverse organizations necessary to achieve equitable, improved treatment. Like a successful venture capital firm, partnerships must effectively orchestrate the resources within and across these organizations . . .[9]

Collaborating in development work has been one approach to interesting the pharmaceutical industry in developing the vaccines needed in poor countries. If companies doubted that they would be able to recoup the vast investments required, they could be given guarantees. This idea has also been followed up through a scheme called the 'Advance Market Commitment'. Widely promoted as an innovative policy mechanism, it is actually comparable with how the National Foundation for Infantile Paralysis had convinced vaccine manufacturers to produce Salk's polio vaccine before it had been proven safe and effective. The Advance Market Commitment (AMC) works through artificially creating a market, provided the new vaccine is developed successfully. There are guarantees to manufacturers, coupled with guarantees of an initially low price to the poor countries, which would form the bulk of the market. If no one is successful in producing the vaccine to predetermined standards, then no public money is spent. With $1.5 billion funding pledged by the Bill and Melinda Gates Foundation and the governments of five donor countries, a pilot AMC was launched in 2009. Its objective was to ensure, and speed up development of, a pneumococcal vaccine that, unlike older pneumococcal vaccines, would be effective in children and which (with the help of additional subsidies) could be introduced in poor countries. The scheme required manufacturers to guarantee the provision of a certain number of doses each year for ten years, at a fixed price of $3.50 per dose, to be topped up to $7 per dose until all the money had been used up. GSK and Pfizer were contracted under the scheme, and they supplied the first of the new 'conjugated' vaccines under the scheme in 2010, the price received being far lower than the price at which they offered the vaccines to industrialized countries. (A 'conjugated' vaccine is one in which a piece of the bacillus is attached to a different, harmless organism in order to trigger a better immune response.) So there is a sense in which the scheme could be regarded as successful, though critics say that the vaccines would have been produced anyway since they were already being developed; that the price of $3.50 is still too high; and that one objective of the scheme (to encourage competition between manufacturers and to encourage manufacturers from the Global South) has certainly not been met.

Emerging Infectious Diseases: A New Concept for Fearful Times

By the start of the new millennium, a few of the IOM's priority vaccines had indeed been developed. There was a hepatitis B vaccine, though this had only been a second order priority in the Institute's view. Higher up the list, there was also a vaccine against rotavirus. However, scientists hadn't yet been able to produce many of those priority vaccines, including a malaria vaccine. From the 1990s onwards, vastly increased sums of money were flowing into malaria-related research, much of it from the u.s. government and from the Bill and Melinda Gates Foundation. Slowly but surely progress was being made. Producing a malaria vaccine poses particular problems because each stage in the parasite's development (known as sporozoites, exoerythrocytic schizonts, merozoites and so on) has different antigens. This implies that a candidate vaccine that protects against one stage probably would not work against another. What is more, not only are the kind of malaria parasites that infect humans different from those that attack other species, so that there's no convenient animal model on which to test candidate vaccines, but they differ from place to place as well. A person who had acquired immunity to the strain in his or her area could well be totally unprotected when exposed to a strain found in a different area. Nevertheless, thanks to new mechanisms for funding, testing and purchasing vaccines, industrial interest was kindled. There are now said to be more than twenty malaria vaccine candidates in clinical development, with GlaxoSmithKline Vaccines' RTS,S already in a large-scale (phase 3) clinical trial. This is the first malaria vaccine candidate to advance this far.

In the meantime, however (and thinking back to the question of whether the many new vaccines reflect new threats to health), one new threat was becoming desperately serious at the time the IOM was writing its report. From 1981 onwards descriptions had begun to accumulate of the disease that later became known as Acquired Immunodeficiency Syndrome, or AIDS. As the nature, extent and severity of what seemed to be a new kind of disease became known, attempts to discover its cause gathered pace. It seemed to strike gay men in particular, and various theories as to why this was were circulating. Moreover, mortality was generally due not to the virus directly, but to some other illness, such as pneumonia, caught as a result of a severely weakened immune system. In 1983 a team led by Luc Montagnier at the Pasteur Institute in Paris identified the virus responsible as belonging to the quite recently discovered family of retroviruses. These viruses consist of RNA rather than DNA and replicate through a different process from other viruses. What Montagnier had found was the virus now known as Human Immunodeficiency Virus-1 (HIV-1), which seemed to have evolved from a virus common in some species of monkey. Following Montagnier's work, and parallel research by Robert Gallo at the American National Cancer Institute, the search for a vaccine began. In 1984, U.S. government representatives announced – with what now seems scarcely credible hubris – that a vaccine should be available for testing in two or three years! Admittedly it was not yet clear if it would be an attenuated- or an inactivated-virus vaccine. The French were less optimistic, and thought it would take longer. In 1986, when the IOM report on vaccine priorities was published, the first AIDS vaccine trials were just starting. No one then suspected how cunning a virus this was. The challenges posed by its ability to hide itself in the body, to attack the immune system, and to replicate and mutate extremely rapidly, were still lying in wait.

Heated discussion of how an HIV vaccine should best be made broke out. Some elder statesmen with long experience of vaccine development (including Jonas Salk) argued that a 'classical' inactivation process offered the simplest route to a vaccine. Stanley Plotkin argued for an attenuated-virus vaccine, though most people thought this too risky. What if an attenuated virus reverted to virulence? However, these approaches had little appeal for the many aggressive newcomers, whose expertise was in genetic engineering. Manipulating genetic material – and not vaccine development – was what Chiron, Genentech, MicroGeneSys, Oncogen, Repligen, and the other biotech firms that soon joined the search for an AIDS vaccine, knew about. The traditional manufacturers were dubious as to whether it would be possible, or what the market would be, and were concerned by the potential liability issues involved. They preferred to invest their resources in developing anti-retroviral drugs, leaving the biotech companies to try to splice genes coding for surface proteins of the HIV virus into some suitable substrate. By the end of the 1980s a number of genetically engineered candidate vaccines were being tried out – not only on animals but also (and despite cries that this was premature and irresponsible) in one or two cases on human volunteers. By 1990 more than twenty AIDS vaccine development projects were under way in the U.S. alone, of which just two were focused on inactivated virus. Deaths from AIDS were rising, but progress was slow, and not only because the science was difficult. The small biotech firms lacked resources and certainly were in no position to mount large-scale clinical trials. Some gave up, while friction between the whole-cell inactivated-vaccine enthusiasts and the genetic engineers continued well into the 1990s. In 1997 President

Clinton announced a commitment to the development of a vaccine within a decade. Once more, many leading scientists thought this foolhardy, doubting that much would even change as a result.

Quite early on, the fundamental question was raised of what a vaccine should be expected to do. A vaccine could be valuable even if it were not able to actually prevent people from becoming infected by the virus. A vaccine could be useful if it simply slowed down the course of the disease: if it was able to decrease the viral load, or 'CD4 count'. But as richer countries began providing anti-retroviral drugs to infected people, how would it be possible to distinguish the effect of the vaccine from those of drugs already in use? Would trials have to be limited to poor countries, where most HIV-infected people still had no access to the fancy new anti-retroviral drugs? This was ethically problematic, since trial participants might be unable to benefit even if the trial was successful and a vaccine developed. The HIV strains circulating differ from place to place. The VaxGen trial that finished in 2003 used slightly different vaccines in its North American and Thai arms, though based on the same concept. It was not deemed to have been successful. Researchers shifted their attention, and a further four trials have been completed. Ideas regarding the kind of vaccine that might ultimately work have been in such flux that some wonder whether a vaccine will ever be possible. A proven vaccine offering significant protection still seems some years in the future.

The Human Immunodeficiency Virus has caused a devastating loss of life, though patients with access to expensive anti-retroviral cocktails no longer live under a death sentence. Obviously the most significant consequence of the HIV epidemic has been the damage it has inflicted on individual lives, on families and communities, and indeed on whole economies, especially in Africa. HIV-infected people are also particularly susceptible to becoming infected by tuberculosis, and paralleling the spread of HIV has been a resurgence of this disease, also claiming millions of lives, and leading to the search for a new and better tuberculosis vaccine. But apart from the lives it claims, directly and indirectly, AIDS has also affected the way infectious disease in general is thought and written about. An earlier optimism, a sense that infectious diseases would soon be wholly controllable, no longer made any sense. In its place came the pervasive sense of threat that films like *Contagion* feed on and into.

In 2014–15, if Western media are any guide, the world's greatest health problem was Ebola. Daily newspaper reports pointed to a growing number of Ebola cases, and more and more deaths. Cases of Ebola were mainly limited to just three desperately poor countries in West Africa, though individual healthcare workers returning to Europe or the u.s. with suspected Ebola got the most publicity. The disease had appeared before. It was first noticed in 1976, when it broke out in Africa and became known as Ebola haemorrhagic fever because one of the outbreaks at that time occurred in a village near the Ebola river, in the Democratic Republic of the Congo. It is now believed that a species of fruit bat is the virus's principal natural host, and that it is introduced into the human population through close contact with the blood, secretions, organs or other bodily fluids of infected animals such as chimpanzees, gorillas, fruit bats, monkeys, forest antelope and porcupines found ill or dead in the forest. The virus is known to be fatal in at least 60 per cent of human cases, and it can now spread from human to human through direct contact with blood or other bodily fluids of infected people, or through contaminated bedding or clothing.

In the 1970s the disease attracted little attention. Then, with the new Ebola epidemic there came a desperate rush to produce a vaccine. How Ebola vaccine development is organized illustrates the complicated arrangements through which health priorities are now translated into research and development projects. In the summer of 2015, promising results were announced of a phase 3 clinical trial of an Ebola vaccine called rvsv-zebov, taking place in Guinea. The trial was funded by the who, with support from the Wellcome Trust, the United Kingdom Department for International Development, the Norwegian Ministry of Foreign Affairs, the Canadian Government and msf. The trial design was developed by a group of experts from Canada, France, Guinea, Norway, Switzerland, the United Kingdom, the United States and the who. The vaccine had originally been developed by scientists working at the Canadian Public Health Agency and was then licensed to a small u.s.-based pharmaceutical company, NewLink genetics. In November 2014, Merck and NewLink Genetics entered into an exclusive world-wide licensing agreement wherein Merck assumed responsibility to research, develop, manufacture and distribute the vaccine that was being investigated. Meanwhile gsk is developing an alternative vaccine in collaboration with the U.S. National Institute of Allergy and Infectious Diseases, while Chinese and Russian investigators are apparently also working on Ebola vaccines. By early 2016 the epidemic had been contained, though at the cost of more than eleven thousand lives, including those of hundreds of African health professionals. As *The Economist* pointed out, the fact that the disease was so serious in the affected countries was due as much to their inadequate health systems as to anything else. The United States, it noted, has 245 doctors per 100,000 people while Guinea, one of the worst affected countries, has only ten. And health professionals were the most likely to succumb and die, adding to the inadequacy of healthcare provision.[10]

AIDS and Ebola are instances of a category that has been pushed to the forefront of international public health discussions: Emerging Infectious Diseases (nowadays known simply as EIDs). With increasing frequency since the 1990s, we have been warned of a whole series of novel threats, some known, others still lurking out there, unknown and mysterious. The wholly unexpected SARS outbreak of 2002–3 (which started in southern China, subsequently spreading to 37 countries and killing nearly eight hundred people) seemed a case in point, as well as seemingly justifying robust global leadership. Like HIV, most new diseases are thought to arise through viruses jumping the species barrier from their normal animal hosts (often bats) and mutating. A term like EID, which lumps together threats of bio-terrorist attacks, of viruses jumping over from the animal kingdom, of diseases reappearing in more virulent form, makes political sense. It holds the attention of media and of politicians. It keeps infectious disease on the health and development agenda and ensures that the money keeps flowing. Despite the huge strides that have been taken in virology and molecular biology, despite all the new vaccines, it is hard to believe that people feel more secure in the face of threats to their health than they did years ago.

Publications of the early 1990s, such as IOM's *Emerging Infections: Microbial Threats to Health in the United States* and Laurie Garrett's bestselling book *The Coming Plague*, gave the concept broad currency. Globalization has made us all so interdependent. It is no longer possible to protect a national population by imposing quarantine at national borders. The extent and speed of mobility, as well as the poor state of disease surveillance in many countries (and sometimes governments' reluctance to admit to the outbreak of an epidemic) have put infectious-disease control near the top of the international agenda. Now deemed too important to be left to ministers of health, infectious-disease control – or 'global health governance' – has become 'securitized'. Increasingly risk-conscious and risk-averse as well, we have largely come to accept that keeping us safe in the face of multiple threats, whether man-made or not, justifies increasingly intrusive surveillance. As citizens, as travellers, we're mostly unaware of what airport body scanners are screening us for: suspicious objects (indicating nefarious intentions) or elevated body temperature (indicating infection)?

Western media seem to discover new epidemics at the rate of one each year. In 2015 it was Ebola that captured media attention, then it was chikungunya in the Caribbean, and in 2016 it was Zika in Latin America. There is no doubting either that these diseases result in death and suffering, or that countless viruses exist that might jump from their animal hosts to infect humans. The concern here is with the lessons that Western media and institutions draw from the suffering of distant people, and the way in which our own fears are nourished and deployed. How much do we read of the environmental conditions – the lack of pure drinking water, the adulterated food, the inadequate or inaccessible health services – that render poor people in Africa, Asia or Latin America so vulnerable to infection? We are encouraged to await development of the vaccine that will solve the problem. As though the mere existence of a vaccine could solve anything! We hear very little about what the vaccine will cost when it has been developed, or how it will be delivered to people who need it most. Of course, those of us who live in what are still relatively rich industrialized countries are also threatened by emerging diseases. But it is by no means obvious that the magnitude of the threat can adequately explain the way in which demand for new vaccines is stimulated or sustained.

Mutating Influenza

Millions of people are advised to have themselves vaccinated against influenza each and every year. Some groups have been identified as being at particular risk of the flu becoming serious, and they are especially targeted. These risk groups, for which many countries provide free vaccinations, include people over 65 years of age and children. In the last few years some countries have followed the lead of the United States and added pregnant women to the list of risk groups for whom flu vaccination is recommended. In fact, since 2010 the CDC has advised that everyone over six months of age should be vaccinated every year against influenza. Clearly this is quite different from the vast majority of vaccines, which are administered just once or twice early in life. How has this come about? Why does a flu jab protect us for just a year? And why are we sometimes warned of especially serious flu epidemics, against which we are advised to take particular precautions?

As we saw in the previous chapter, by the late 1940s it was known that the influenza virus mutates. It followed that, to be effective, vaccines would have to be adjusted in the light of circulating (sub-) strains. By 1950 the WHO had established an international network of specialized public health laboratories, now known as the Global Influenza Surveillance and Response System (GISRS). Since the 1970s one responsibility of this network has been to gather samples of circulating influenza viruses each year, and to identify those that may pose the greatest risk. Vaccine candidate strains are then sent to vaccine manufacturers for production of seasonal influenza vaccines. Prior to recent objections from developing-country vaccine manufacturers, these were all located in industrialized countries. There is usually little time – a few months – between delivery of the year's virus strains and the onset of the seasonal influenza epidemic when the vaccine would be needed.

Compared to the 1940s, when the first influenza vaccines were developed, a great deal more is known about the virus today. It is known that influenza type A (but not B or C) can infect other animal species in addition to humans: notably fowl and other birds, pigs, dogs and horses. All three types are made of segments of genetic material contained in a shell consisting of two surface proteins, haemagglutinin (H) and neuraminidase (N). The genes that relate to these proteins are constantly mutating, with the result that the virus's outer surface looks different, and antibodies that protected against a previous infection can no longer do their job. This so-called 'antigenic drift' is only part of what makes it all so tricky. More fundamental mutations (known as 'antigenic shift') take place when a type A strain affecting another species (such as pigs or birds) jumps the species barrier as a result of close human contact with infected animals. This doesn't happen easily. Another danger is that the bird or pig flu virus exchanges genetic material with the flu virus of another species, resulting in a new flu type, with a different H and N shell, against which humans may have little protection. If the new flu type spreads easily from person to person, then a pandemic may occur.

Panic broke out in the United States in 1976 because a u.s. army recruit was found to be infected by an H1N1 influenza virus closely related to the one that had caused the 1918 epidemic. This was the 'swine flu': the epidemic-that-never-was mentioned earlier, from which only one person died.

In 2003–5 the avian flu epidemic (with a different protein shell, known as H5N1), provoked panicked reactions. As its name suggests, it is carried by birds: rarely pet birds, parrots or pigeons; more usually chickens and other farm birds that become infected and can pass on the virus. The H5N1 virus seems to infect more species than any previously known influenza virus and is continuing to evolve. Most cases of infection occurred in South and Southeast Asia. Although millions of birds have become infected with the virus since its discovery, human deaths have been limited since the virus is not easily transmitted from one human to another. Some 359 people, spread over twelve countries, are believed to have died from the H5N1 virus. Avian influenza vaccines have been prepared and licensed but are not in widespread use.

In recent years, there have been more and more warnings that a pandemic as deadly as that of 1918 is imminent. In 2009 H1N1, the strain that really worries virologists, returned. Though it was an H1N1 virus, it was not identical to the H1N1 virus involved in the 1976 'epidemic'. Analysis showed that it was a new strain of H1N1, formed by an existing blend (the proper term is 'reassortment') of bird, swine and human flu viruses, further combined with a pig flu virus, thus leading to the term 'swine flu'. The virus seems to have emerged in Veracruz, in Mexico, which is why it also acquired the name 'Mexican flu'. The Mexican government closed down most of the city's public facilities in an attempt to halt the spread of the virus, but it nevertheless spread around the world. Unlike most strains of influenza, and to the surprise of epidemiologists, this virus was found disproportionately to infect younger adults rather than the elderly. In June 2009 the WHO declared the outbreak to be a pandemic. This decision was based not on advice from its permanent vaccine advisory committee (known as the Strategic Advisory Group of Experts, or SAGE), but on the advice of an emergency committee, the names of whose members were not made public at the time. The announcement of a pandemic automatically triggered the conditional orders for vaccine that rich countries had already placed with vaccine manufacturers. The governments of many European countries ordered two doses for every inhabitant, amounting to hundreds of millions of doses, costing hundreds of millions of euros. Fortunately, or unfortunately, by the time the bulk of the vaccine orders had been delivered the number of cases was already tapering off. In the summer of 2010 the WHO announced that the pandemic had ended. The virus had been far less deadly than experts had predicted. Estimates of how many people died from this H1N1 epidemic vary widely (from ten thousand to some hundreds of thousands) and have been disputed. What does seem clear is that most deaths occurred not in Europe but in Africa and Southeast Asia. In the event, most of the vaccine was unused, as it had been bought by the world's more affluent countries and had often arrived when the epidemic was past its high point. Countries that had not been able to push themselves to the front of the queue no longer had an interest in purchasing surplus vaccine. Millions of doses, which would be of no value in combatting a future influenza epidemic (and which some critics claimed had not been properly tested for safety) had to be destroyed.

Fierce debate followed, with critics claiming that the WHO had exaggerated the danger, spreading 'fear and confusion' rather than 'immediate information'. Committees of enquiry were appointed to investigate decision-making at the WHO and national levels. On what basis, and on whose advice, had the pandemic been declared? On what basis and on whose advice had national health authorities signed secret contracts with multinational vaccine manufacturers? When it finally became known that many of the most influential advisers, at both WHO and national levels, were paid consultants to the vaccine industry, many commentators were appalled. Whose interests had they been serving? Wasn't this a clear case of conflict of interests?

Dynamics of the Global Vaccine Market

The global vaccine market has an incredible dynamic. The amount of money spent on purchasing vaccines, globally, is said to have risen from $5 billion in 2000 to almost $24 billion by 2013 and is forecast to reach $100 billion by 2025.[11] How is this to be explained? By the discovery of new pathogens and the introduction of vaccines against EIDs? There is no doubt that a great deal of attention is going to the EIDs. Partly, without question, because large-scale and rapid population movements now spread diseases originating in animals around the world: diseases which might once have remained confined to remote villages. There are new threats, but few of these vaccines are yet licensed and in use. Is the growth of the market due to more vaccination in the developing world? We will discuss this later, but I think the tentative answer is 'only to a limited extent'. Crucially, what was once an underdeveloped segment within the pharmaceutical industry has now become the vehicle for its further growth, with no less than 120 new vaccine products said to be in the development pipeline. If these new vaccines are to recoup their development costs, demand for them will have to be created. One way in which this is being done is by making us – people living in the world's rich countries – more risk-averse, more risk-conscious and more fearful of potential risks to our health. While we've been waiting for the most-needed vaccines, such as those against HIV and malaria, we have been provided with a number of others, offering protection against diseases that we had previously thought inconsequential. Chickenpox, or varicella, is an example.

Because of the lesions it produces, chickenpox was once thought to be a mild form of smallpox. In fact it is caused by a quite different virus, now known as the varicella zoster virus, a form of herpes virus. Chickenpox is something that almost all children used to catch. It is very contagious, spread through the air by coughs and sneezes, but rarely serious. Its characteristic itchy and unpleasant rash generally clears up after a week or so. Complications are rare in children (though more common in adults who catch the disease for the first time), and only a small number of infected children require hospital care. However, once symptoms have disappeared the virus can remain dormant in the body, emerging many years later, especially in people with compromised immune systems, as shingles (also known as herpes zoster). A varicella vaccine was produced in Japan, in the mid-1970s, by attenuating live virus taken from an infected child. It was first used in an Osaka hospital to prevent children infecting one another. This so-called Oka strain later became the basis for vaccine trials carried out in the 1980s, and led to vaccines produced and marketed by Merck (starting in 1995), by GSK, and by Biken (in Japan).

Since parents in North America, Australia and Western Europe mostly didn't think of chickenpox as anything other than a normal childhood affliction that would go away by itself in a few days, it was not obvious that there would be any demand for a vaccine. In fact, though it was soon made a routine vaccination in the U.S. and Canada, in other countries (including Japan, where it was first developed) its introduction has been slow. Even now most European countries have not introduced it routinely. But in the United States two kinds of argument were used to help create a market. One was economic. Estimates of the costs of chickenpox, to the family and to the state, could be set against the cost of vaccination. Provided the costs resulting from a sick child were defined widely enough (so not just the costs of doctors and medicines, but indirect costs such as the five or six working days that parents might lose, or school-days lost, or extra babysitting) then the vaccine could be shown to be cost-effective. Second, the disease was made to seem less mild than most people thought, by emphasizing the number of deaths attributed to it. Of the four million or so cases each year in the United States, in pre-vaccine days, there were 100–150 deaths annually. Expressed as a percentage of the number of people affected, the death rate (less than 0.004 per cent) is obviously far too small to cause much anxiety. But people would react differently if told that each year more than a hundred people died of chickenpox. Later, concerns emerged that immunity might decline with the passage of time, leading to the risk of infection being postponed to older ages – at which infection with shingles carries greater risk. The solution first proposed was a second dose of the vaccine, but now there is a new vaccine for adults at risk of becoming infected.

The market for an 'orphan vaccine' can also be enhanced by combining it with one that is widely used, as was done with the mumps vaccine long ago. More recently both Merck and GSK have combined varicella vaccine with the measles-mumps-rubella (MMR) vaccine, which is a mainstay of vaccine programmes in almost all industrialized countries. Both companies' four-component (tetravalent) vaccines were licensed in the USA in 2006. If these two companies, with their vast shares of the vaccine market, were to offer only the tetravalent product, and to no longer offer MMR, then countries with little interest in chickenpox vaccination would have no option but to use it.

As scientists learn more and more about how the immune system works, new vistas, new challenges, the possibility of vaccines against conditions or behaviours that have nothing to do with infectious disease open up. At present, based on new insights from immunology, considerable research is being devoted to the search for cancer vaccines. Of course a vaccine against the human papilloma virus, which may lead to cervical cancer, has existed for some years. But since this virus is mainly transmitted through sexual contact, it is also an infectious disease and thus somewhat different from cancers arising in totally different ways. There is now a decade of work aimed at developing vaccines that should help the body resist or slow down tumour growth, and a few of these vaccines are the subject of clinical trials. For example, early stage (phase 1 or 2) clinical trials of breast cancer vaccines and lung cancer vaccines are currently under way.

Scientists are also investigating how stress influences immunity to infection, and how immunity influences behaviour. A whole new field of scientific research, known as psychoneuroimmunology, is opening up, the implications of which are now a matter for excited speculation. It is starting to seem as though any physical or mental condition that is frightening, needlessly risky, or socially unacceptable is a potential focus for vaccine development. Cancer isn't the only area of non-infectious disease control that has sparked the search for a vaccine. Contraception is another. The idea of immunological contraception isn't wholly new, though in recent years a number of different approaches have been developed. Some of these are now used as an alternative to castration of pets and farm animals. The basic idea is that the immune system is used to prevent fertilization, or to prevent implantation of an embryo. People working in the field seem to regard immuno-contraception as preferable to existing methods because it could have various applications. Vaccines based upon reproductive hormones could be used for reversible contraception, for permanent sterilization, for delaying sexual maturation, for blocking hormone-dependent tumours or for combatting hormone-expressing tumours.

As far as use in humans is concerned – and they could be available for both men and women – contraceptive vaccines are still in the experimental stage. So too are vaccines against nicotine addiction. The rationale here, of course, is that quitting smoking is difficult. Existing 'treatments' aren't very effective. What's more, smoking endangers the health not only of the smoker but also of people passively exposed to cigarette smoke. The principle of an anti-smoking vaccine is to induce antibodies that would bind the nicotine in the blood, so preventing it from crossing the blood–brain barrier. It is because of the way that the nicotine acts on the brain that smoking is addictive. The nicotine molecule isn't capable of inducing antibodies, so in experimental vaccines it is attached ('conjugated') to a carrier protein. A number of anti-smoking vaccines are being developed by various biotechnology companies, though none is anywhere near licensing. Further in the future, but nevertheless being discussed, are vaccines against obesity and even depression.

The search for new ways of delivering vaccines adds further dynamics to the vaccine field. Many people, especially children, don't like needles being stuck into them. The fact that it was given orally, on a sugar cube, was seen as making Sabin's polio vaccine more acceptable to parents than Salk's vaccine that was injected. Since then, an influenza vaccine given through a nasal spray in place of a needle, first developed in Russia, has become widely used. Edible vaccines are still under development. Potatoes, bananas, rice and other plants have been genetically modified so as to express surface antigens from the hepatitis B virus, for example. Remember, there are currently something like seven hundred vaccine-related clinical trials!

Tensions in the System

Why are there more and more vaccines? Are they the ones we – but then who are 'we'? – most need or most want? Or put differently, how far – and how – is vaccine development responding to public health need?

Looking back, it is clear that the way in which vaccines are conceived, developed and produced has changed vastly from the early days. A hundred years ago, as the bacterial causes of diseases such as diphtheria, tuberculosis, typhoid and typhus were identified – diseases responsible for terrible loss of life – discoveries triggered attempts at developing vaccines against them. Of course there were many failures. Some diseases, caused by what would later come to be known as viruses, proved recalcitrant. A crucial step in producing a vaccine is harvesting a sufficient supply of the pathogen, and viruses could not be grown in the usual way. Sometimes there were difficulties in scaling up production, or in deciding between different ways of inactivating or attenuating the pathogen. Ways of standardizing quality and potency had to be developed, as did procedures for imposing these standards on producers. The early vaccines were largely produced in institutions attached in one way or another to local or national departments of health. Their vaccine production reflected public health doctors' assessment of need – though doctors in private practice didn't necessarily agree. Communities may have been resistant, and (as we will soon see) the very idea of using vaccines for public health goals was more enthusiastically received in some states than in others. The model – vaccine producers linked to public health institutions and concerns – was exported through colonial administrations, through the network of Pasteur Institutes, and through the work of the Rockefeller Foundation in Latin America. At the same time in some countries – Germany, the United Kingdom and the United States among them – private pharmaceutical companies were becoming an important, and very soon the principal, source of vaccines. Though only very gradually, commercial considerations would lead to attenuation of the link between producers and public health authorities. Still, until well after the Second World War, with production of new viral vaccines – polio, measles, influenza – in full swing, there was little sign of what this would later imply. But at the same time, pharmaceutical companies brought new resources and a new dynamism into the field.

Like all medical technologies, vaccines have a dual identity. For ministries of health, for public health practitioners, for physicians and nurses, they are above all tools of public health: tools with which they can protect the health of their patients and of their communities. Despite their inefficiency and (in some cases) lack of resources, this held for the public-sector vaccine institutes that once met a large proportion of the world's demand for vaccines.

It was to some degree also true of the long-established vaccine manufacturers, though these necessarily sought ways of reconciling their obligations in the public sphere with their need to invest their resources profitably. The private manufacturers prior to the 1980s, producing largely for national or regional markets, were able to maintain good relations with the public health officials who were their customers.

In the 1970s some companies had second thoughts. Vaccines were more difficult to make than pharmaceuticals and less profitable, and since they were intended for millions of healthy babies the implications of something going wrong were horrendous. A suggestion that the whooping cough vaccine might cause neurological damage was the final straw for some. Many abandoned vaccine production, to the consternation of public health officials in the United States in particular.

Starting in the 1980s, just as new ways of making vaccines were developed, knowledge was increasingly privatized. In the neo-liberal era the public-sector vaccine institutes that remained found their access to 'intellectual property' barred by patents and by legislation and international treaties. Allowing free play to market forces came to seem the only way of doing almost everything. As 'shareholder value' was increasingly prioritized, interests began to move further and further apart. Industry, increasingly oriented to profit-maximization, had no interest whatever in developing vaccines only needed in countries that would be unable to pay for them. Even now there are no vaccines against the parasitic diseases schistosomiasis (or bilharzia), transmitted by snails, or leishmaniasis (or kala azar), carried by sandflies, each of which affect millions of people in tropical and subtropical regions. Their importance from a public health perspective is clear, but without a major source of subsidy it would be impossible for the costs of development and production to be recouped through commercial sales. The pharmaceutical industry isn't really interested. The divergence of public health from industrial priorities, with the key decisions regarding which vaccines were to be developed being taken by corporate management, was noted with anxiety in the public health world.

The relative importance of the needs (and market appeal) of rich and poor countries is illustrated by the history of a vaccine called RotaShield, developed by Wyeth and licensed in the USA in

1998. Diarrhoeal disease is common and often severe among children living in areas lacking good-quality drinking water. Rotavirus infection is the source of a particularly dangerous form of diarrhoea, and the Institute of Medicine had seen development of a rotavirus vaccine as a high priority. The pathogen had been identified by researchers at the Royal Children's Hospital in Melbourne in 1973. Trials had shown that RotaShield conferred 50–60 per cent protection against all cases of rotavirus diarrhoea, and 70–100 per cent protection against severe disease. Uptake in the USA was rapid, and within the course of nine months some 600,000 infants had received the vaccine. However, by July 1999, fifteen cases of intussusception, a rare but potentially fatal blockage of the intestine, were reported to the country's adverse-events reporting system (known by the acronym VAERS). Further cases in vaccine recipients were reported thereafter, and a causal link between intussusception and the vaccine seemed probable. Although estimates of the risk of this severe adverse event varied widely, in October 1999 the U.S. Advisory Committee on Immunization Practices and the CDC withdrew their recommendation for RotaShield and the manufacturer voluntarily stopped producing it. Internationally, this decision came in for some criticism, since this was the only licensed rotavirus vaccine. Critics argued that it deprived children in the developing world, for whom rotavirus infection presents a far greater risk than it did in the U.S., of a potentially life-saving innovation. Fortunately by 2005 other rotavirus vaccines had become available.

Vaccines are not tools of public health alone. From another perspective they are potentially profitable commodities. Modern vaccines are products that make use of highly sophisticated science and technology, difficult and expensive to develop, and potentially very profitable. The biotech companies that, from the 1980s, saw vaccine development as a potentially fruitful area for deploying the expertise over which they had a virtual monopoly, had no history of public health involvement. Reflecting the very different nature of these companies, the growing role of venture capital, and the growing emphasis on maximizing shareholders' return on investment, the vaccine industry was changing. From a company's perspective it made economic sense to develop any vaccine for which a market could be established in the industrialized world. The trick then would be gaining the influence needed, whether over public health policymakers or the population at large, for an effective demand to emerge. The objective would have to be to convince the world that if a vaccine could be made, it should be used: that any threat, or potential threat, that could in principle be reduced by vaccination was worth the effort. Why let your child run any risk at all? Just as healthcare in general isn't any longer limited to curing disease, so the scope of vaccination is being extended far beyond the prevention of life-threatening infectious diseases. Where once vaccine development took its priorities from what were clearly major threats to the health of the community, this is no longer wholly the case. Popular, and indeed political, perceptions of common conditions are malleable. They can be influenced, with the result that we are led to fear illnesses that our parents used to view with a resigned shrug of the shoulders.

In the last thirty years the link between vaccine development and public health concerns has changed. This is not to say that there is no such link. The innovation system still seeks to respond rapidly to threats, or what can appear as threats. Threats to what? As much as by the well-being of their citizens, countries of the Global North are concerned by perceived biological threats to their national security. Vaccines are developed with these threats in mind, rather than the much greater public health need in countries whose ability to pay is doubtful. Admittedly, donor and philanthropic funds, and new incentives and mechanisms, have brought more attention to healthcare technologies designed specifically for use in developing countries. And at the same time manufacturers in India and other developing countries, growing in size and now organized in a Developing Countries Vaccine Manufacturers' Network, may well bring about a further change in the dynamic of the system.

The future of the vaccine enterprise will continue to depend on careful tailoring of publicity. There has to be a sense of threat: a latent sense of lurking pathogens waiting to attack us. We mustn't feel too safe. On the other hand, if public health authorities cry wolf too often there is a risk of confidence being undermined.

FIVE

POLICIES:
HESITANT BEGINNINGS

Public Health Technologies

What exactly are vaccines? We saw earlier that from a biomedical perspective their defining characteristic is that vaccines are 'immunogenic'. That is to say, they stimulate the body's immune system to respond to an attack. The biomedical literature is filled with studies of the body's immune system, and with discussion of how vaccines work. Today, as we have just seen, there are attempts to develop vaccines against health risks quite different from the ones posed by infectious diseases. Few people seem to be aware of the effort going into the development of breast cancer vaccines, or contraceptive vaccines, or anti-smoking vaccines. Most of us think of vaccines in terms of infectious-disease prevention. Although the range of vaccines offered to teenagers is growing, and older people are encouraged to go for a flu jab every year, small children are the major focus of vaccination efforts. Vaccines are different from drugs not only because they are (or at least used to be) prepared from dangerous germs, but also because they are given to healthy, not sick, people. A healthy European baby will receive something like ten different antigens before it reaches its first birthday, with more to follow. The expectation is that all children will be vaccinated, and in the industrialized world most are. Indeed in some countries vaccination is compulsory, so that a child that hasn't been fully vaccinated might be forbidden to go to school, or its parents might be denied child benefit. As movies like *Contagion* show so vividly, the threat of an epidemic pushes the vaccine development system into overdrive. Laboratories work day and night trying to develop, test and produce the vaccine as rapidly as possible. In a public health emergency, there may be some relaxation of the time-consuming tests required before a vaccine can be licensed for widespread use. Governments jostle to position themselves at the head of the queue for when it becomes available. When there is an epidemic, and all eyes are fixed on them, ministers of health try to reassure people that they are doing everything possible to provide the necessary drugs, vaccines or facilities. Under more normal circumstances, when there is no epidemic, a different kind of rationality is at play. Because immunization is now a key – perhaps *the* key – component of preventive health, we would expect policies to be subject to careful scrutiny. That should mean not only that people are convinced that there is a threat to their health but also that there is robust evidence for the safety and the efficacy of the vaccines.

When it has been decided that a new antigen is to be added to the national immunization programme, the population will be given estimates of the number of lives that will be saved, or the number of cases of severe diarrhoea, or cervical cancer, or sensory impairment that will be prevented. In the decision-making process, cost–benefit calculations are likely to have played an important role, but these won't be publicized as widely. Depending on the way government works in one country or another, vaccination policies may be debated, subject to discussion about the numbers, the details, the costs and the possible side effects. However, the general idea that the goal of vaccination is to save lives (rather than money) and to prevent needless illness, dominates popular thinking. It underpins the numbers that are routinely collected; numbers showing huge decreases in mortality from smallpox, diphtheria, yellow fever, polio and many more diseases after the start of mass vaccination.

Instead of thinking about vaccines in terms of what makes them distinctive, we can also think about them as a particular type of 'public health technology'. There are many technologies for protecting the health of the population, ranging from water purification to bed nets, and from vitamin supplements to genetic screening, so that vaccines lose their uniqueness. Technologies are tools, devices that in one way or another enhance what we are able to do, singly or collectively. Most technologies enable us to do things that we could do before, but in ways that we regard as 'better'. 'Better' might mean faster, or more safely, or more cheaply, or more efficiently: it depends on the kind of activity involved. Engineers developing and designing new or improved technologies have to make all kinds of choices. What do customers want, and how much will they be willing to pay for it? Should the aim be greater speed or safety, or should it be lower cost? Outward appearances notwithstanding, there is nothing 'inevitable' in the way in which technologies evolve. Everything depends on the choices being made, and these in turn depend on their developers' or manufacturers' assessment of the interests, skills and resources of potential users. Sometimes distinctive market segments with different preferences emerge, as with automobiles. Because the market is so large, different models can be produced for groups with different priorities: fast sports cars for some, suvs for others, and solid economical family cars for yet others. But the markets for nuclear power stations, or anti-missile defence systems, or telephone exchanges, aren't like that. There may be not only competing products to be considered, but also competing technologies. Nuclear power stations compete with coal-fired ones, as well as with solar panels and wind turbines. It's no different with medical technologies. When the first MRI scanners were approaching production, their manufacturers had to think not only about what hospitals and radiologists wanted, but also about satisfying the regulatory agencies (notably the Food and Drug Administration, or FDA). They would have to compete with each other, but they shared an interest in proving that the new technology offered benefits over the previous new scanning technology (CT) in which hospitals had recently made large investments.

It is difficult to predict exactly what a new technology will do, despite all the effort that has gone into trying. Many complications make prediction difficult. One is scale effects. Having a telephone, when only very few people had them, may have been fun, and it may have been a mark of distinction. But its transformative effect on people's lives only emerged later, as almost everyone acquired one and almost everyone could be telephoned. At the same time, with the growing scale of production, costs should (in principle) fall so that more people have access. Perhaps the biggest difficulty comes from the fact that new technologies almost always have effects other than that for which they were developed. To start with, there is little incentive for anyone to look far beyond the ostensible purpose of the technology. When it arrived, the automobile offered a liberating experience for its owners: freedom of movement, speed, independence. This is how potential customers were expected to think of it. And of course they did. Only science fiction writers imagined some of the effects of large-scale automobile use that emerged later: deaths in traffic accidents (a leading cause of death in some parts of the world), air pollution and the environmental and geopolitical effects of demand for oil. In the case of medical technologies, including vaccines, increasingly stringent regulations require careful reporting of any side effects before the vaccine or drug can be licensed for use. But even so, assumptions have to be made about what side effects to look for. Side effects can only be studied when means exist of doing so. For example, the scope for ascertaining the effect of a drug or a surgical intervention on brain activity was limited before brain-imaging technologies had been developed. So it happens that doubts can emerge long after a medical technology has entered widespread use. The claim that the pertussis vaccine could lead to brain damage (later shown to be unfounded) emerged thirty years after its introduction.

Interlocking interests and mutual interdependencies emerge around technologies. Car use sustains not only the automobile industry (while leaving abandoned sites of production to decay as it relocates), but also distributors, tyre manufacturers, the oil industry, garages and pump stations, automobile associations and schools of mechanical engineering. Though each has a vested interest in automobile use, its significance for each is different. A consequence is that they will look quite differently at potentially game-changing developments like, for example, electric cars. For reasons similarly based in interests or ideology, what seems to one group to be convincing evidence for the dramatic consequences of (for example) fossil fuel consumption, is dismissed by its opponents. Disagreement about the significance of scientific evidence isn't limited to public controversies such as those around climate change or the dangers of fracking. It is actually quite common in science and in medicine, where different specializations look at phenomena differently. It sometimes happens that clinicians are convinced by a few cases of spectacular recovery that epidemiologists find statistically meaningless. There is no position of superior rationality from which we can say that one perspective is more valid than the other.

Uncertainties, unpredictability, unintended consequences and potentially conflicting perspectives are all inherent to the process of technological change. The kind of evidence that convinces – whether about climate change or anything else – will reflect the current state of play in often invisible power struggles.

Because the majority of people living in the industrialized world now take vaccines so much for granted, mainstream media do not normally discuss them as one form of public health technology among many. Accounts of vaccine development generally emphasize continuing success in the conquest of infectious diseases: the number of lives saved, the diseases that have been rendered 'vaccine-preventable'. Of course this is perfectly legitimate. There can be no questioning of the fact that vaccines have made it possible vastly to reduce the numbers of people dying from infectious diseases, just as automobiles have enabled many people to move around more conveniently. However, thinking of vaccines not as something *sui generis* but as *technologies* for protecting public health, leads to new questions.

The technologies that researchers try to develop and that entrepreneurs try to bring to the market reflect perceptions both of scientific feasibility and of need or potential demand. Decisions about the investment of resources always involve these two sorts of consideration, in one mix or another. When the u.s. Institute of Medicine tried to develop a blueprint for vaccine futures, in 1984, it looked both at feasibility and at need. But when epidemiologists, or immunologists, or pharmaceutical company executives think about a 'better' vaccine, the chances are they have quite different possibilities in mind. What makes one vaccine against a particular disease better than another? Some will be thinking in technical terms: a different preservative or adjuvant, or enhanced thermal stability. A global effort to eradicate smallpox could only succeed because the Russians had developed freeze-dried vaccine. The liquid vaccine used in the West was not stable enough in tropical climates. Greater safety is an increasingly important incentive. Recombinant hepatitis B vaccine was developed to replace the earlier plasma-derived vaccine because it promised to eliminate any risk of HIV contamination. The acellular pertussis vaccine was developed and introduced because it promised to assuage the fears of parents, worried by research (dramatized by the media) suggesting that the older whole cell vaccine could damage their child's brain. The new vaccine was much more expensive and later appeared to protect for significantly fewer years than the older vaccine. If the focus had been on keeping cost down or on duration of protection, then perhaps the acellular vaccine would never have been developed. Apart from scientific or technical feasibility, vaccine development responds to changes in the world in which we live. Trench warfare in 1914–18 added urgency to the search for a typhoid vaccine. Climate change seems to threaten the temperate north with malaria. Population movements and collapsing health services add urgency to the search for a better vaccine against tuberculosis, which again threatens the industrialized world. Globalization puts people in Amsterdam, London or New York at risk from new diseases originating in animals and emerging in regions that are no longer so remote.

Public health isn't much served by the mere existence of a new vaccine. Political decisions regarding its use will have to be taken. Vaccination policy involves decisions about the introduction of new antigens into vaccination programmes, about payments and compulsions, about how to extend coverage in under-vaccinated communities, or about meeting targets agreed in Geneva or New York. These decisions might be based on epidemiological data, or on public demand, protest or resistance. They might be based on pressure from the country's medical profession or from pharmaceutical companies, or they might be a response to emerging international consensus or pressure. The governments of poor countries, some of which depend on donor aid for keeping even basic health services going, cannot afford to ignore what international agencies and donors recommend. Having taken the decision to extend coverage or introduce a new vaccine, that vaccine will have to be acquired. Perhaps an international organization such as UNICEF can help to obtain it cheaply. Then there will have to be ways of distributing it, and if it deteriorates easily in a tropical climate (as many vaccines do), refrigeration technology, a so-called 'cold chain', will be needed. Actually administering the vaccine may involve government health workers, pharmacies, general practitioners, well-baby clinics, nurses, lay vaccinators and, possibly, mobile health centres. Do parents want to have their children vaccinated? If there is an epidemic, or they have been told that one is coming, there will probably be widespread demand for the new vaccine, or disputes over who should have priority if there isn't enough to go round. On the other hand, when a disease isn't perceived as very threatening, or when it is perceived as being due to supernatural causes, there might be indifference or even reluctance to make the effort. Parents will have to be encouraged, or induced, to go along to the clinic, to their GP, or to the mobile vaccination unit when it turns up in their village. Public health authorities may have to resort to publicity campaigns, or to dream up incentives, to encourage vaccination. Or they may dream up coercions or punishments for those who resist persuasion, as they did with compulsory smallpox vaccination in the nineteenth century, and have done again, much more recently.

In previous chapters we saw how social and political changes, changing configurations of interests, resources and authority have influenced where, how and against what vaccines are developed and produced. The policies and practices involved in getting vaccines out into the community have also responded to social and political changes. It seems reasonable to expect changes in government ideology or social values to impact more directly on vaccine policies than on the development and production of vaccines. The entrepreneurs and industrial executives whose decisions have become decisive for vaccine development are responsible to their shareholders, to 'the market'. They are well aware that they will be held accountable on the basis of the return on investment they give or promise their shareholders, or the company's share of what is now a global market. In principle at least, ministers of health and their officials are responsible to their citizens, and might expect to be judged – among other things – on the basis of adequacy of and access to healthcare. Increasingly, however, as we will see, health officials are made responsible to the international community, bound either by requirements imposed on them by donors, or by international health agreements. What pharmaceutical industry executives and public health officials have in common is that both face a growing emphasis on demonstrating success. An effective vaccine, widely used, can help both of them meet their needs.

So in this and the following two chapters we turn back in order to tell a different story. It is a more complex one, a more difficult story to tell than the vaccine-development story, because there is less of an intuitive sense of progress, of linearity. For something like two hundred years the view of science as constant progress, improvement and advance has been cemented into Western culture, with only the occasional critic gaining much of an audience.

In previous chapters I have tried to tell the story of vaccine development, which of course has drawn on the sciences of bacteriology, virology and immunology, in a way that isn't wholly subordinated to the dominant narrative of progress. When we turn to look at how vaccines have been made use of, and deployed in the interest of public health, a notion of progress is less all-pervasive. Of course numbers – lives saved by vaccinations, or impairments prevented – are used to construct such an account, but this has much shallower roots. Moreover, as we will see later, it is far more widely contested. This has to be a story of diversity, since the politics surrounding vaccination programmes will somehow reflect national political differences and divisions. We'd expect vaccination programmes to differ from country to country, depending at least on the burden of disease, the wealth of the country, the organization of healthcare, and the ideological complexion of its government. And to start with, as vaccines were gradually acknowledged as a potentially valuable tool of public health, their use did indeed differ greatly from one country to another.

Protecting Communities and Protecting Trade

There was growing attention for public health in the course of the nineteenth century. National and local governments concerned themselves increasingly with the health of people living within their borders or representing their interests abroad. Many influences pushed them into doing so, among them religiously inspired philanthropy, fears that epidemic disease could lead to a breakdown in the social order, and the wish to protect commercial interests. As public health became a field of state action, in the mid-nineteenth century, vaccines were of limited importance in the overall scheme of things. Many of the diseases that would later come to be regarded as 'vaccine-preventable' were more or less indistinguishable, since they could only be diagnosed on the basis of symptoms and these often overlapped. Depending upon what were thought to be the causes and mode of transmission of disease, as well as on political and administrative traditions, practice in some places emphasized sanitary measures, while in others it emphasized restrictions on mobility such as quarantine. In so far as infectious disease was thought to be caused by filth, by insanitary and unhygienic living conditions (especially marked, of course, among people living in poverty), sanitary inspection and improvement made sense. In so far as it was thought to be the result of contagion, restrictions on the movement of people, but also movement of ships and possibly of goods that might harbour an infectious agent (bales of cotton, for example, or wool), made sense. In some places, at some times, one approach dominated. In other places, at other times, the other. By the time diphtheria antitoxin became widely available, public health had developed its own ways of doing things: practices that differed from place to place, but all intended to reduce the collective risk of infectious disease. These established public health practices provided the background to the deployment of the new sera and vaccines.

Britain in the 1840s and '50s was particularly committed to a sanitationist approach. Infectious disease was the result of the unhygienic living conditions so powerfully evoked by Friedrich Engels. Putrefying organic matter produced the 'morbid atmosphere' that bred disease. The dominant view was that while quarantine could hinder transmission, only sanitary measures could eliminate the cause. Legislation of 1848 established a General Board of Health, as well as local boards of health that in turn appointed their own medical officers of health. The responsibilities of the local boards focused mainly on sanitary issues, and they had the right to force house owners to improve the sanitary condition of their properties. In other countries, contagionist views held sway, and more emphasis was placed on preventing contact between infected and non-infected people. Over time, new knowledge (as well as new threats) led to modifications of established practices. Long before Koch identified the comma bacillus as the cause of cholera, it was becoming clear to many that cholera epidemics came from the Orient, and that new modes of transportation (steamships, railways) were facilitating its spread. Contagion was obviously involved, whatever the role of local sanitary conditions, and there was a clear need to impose quarantine. On the other hand, applying the same measures indiscriminately on all traffic from the East would be costly. There were objections, both from merchants whose business would be disrupted and from advocates of free trade. A more selective approach to quarantine, designating certain points of departure as 'risky', could provoke countermeasures from countries that were singled out. But failure to introduce quarantine could also lead to tensions with neighbouring countries. It was not only the fear of cholera that provoked such debates. Yellow fever, coming from the West this time, posed another terrifying threat. By the 1870s, people living in West Africa, in the Caribbean, in Buenos Aires and Rio de Janeiro, and in cities on the east coast of the United States, were well aware of what a yellow fever epidemic could do. Everywhere, quarantine was a sensitive and controversial topic, often pitting commercial interests against public opinion. The controversy led to a need to establish more precisely what or who had to be quarantined. Techniques of inspection and surveillance were needed, so that restrictions could be limited to individuals found to be infected. Before vaccines were ever made, it was in this area that bacteriology yielded its early benefits. In 1883 Koch announced that he had succeeded in identifying the cause of cholera. Though it would be years before there would be an effective cholera vaccine, Koch's discovery meant that people who would need to be quarantined could be identified not only by symptoms (which could easily be confused with those of other gastric illnesses), but by the presence of the bacillus. Koch's discovery influenced and was integrated into, but certainly did not displace, existing methods of protecting public health.

By the time the first new sera and vaccines became available, many countries already had some years of experience with smallpox vaccination. Its unpopularity was due in part to the procedure. This involved repeatedly scraping the arm with a special pointed tool to break the skin, after which the lymph was applied. Often it was badly done by unskilled vaccinators, leaving people with nasty scars. Countries that had started mass smallpox vaccination had had to create administrative structures for carrying it out. In England the system was administered by the Poor Law Guardians – another reason for its unpopularity there. In 1853 smallpox vaccination was made compulsory in England, and parents or guardians who failed to vaccinate a child in its first three months of life became liable to a fine or imprisonment. The incidence of smallpox was being brought down, but the processes and practices involved were hugely unpopular. A number of influential people also spoke out publicly against compulsory vaccination, either because of their contagionist views (as was the case with Herbert Spencer) or because they opposed involvement of the state in the field of health. Somewhat similar systems were put in place in other European countries. In the Netherlands, despite the objections of strongly Protestant communities, an 1872 law required proof of vaccination before a child could be admitted to school. The rate of vaccination rose to some 90 per cent, though here too the procedure remained highly unpopular. In parts of pre-unification Germany there had been a longer acknowledgement that the health of the population was a responsibility of the state. In Prussia, a system of local government vaccinators had been established, and here too vaccination was free for the poor. However, informed opinion gradually began to favour general compulsion, and in 1874 an Imperial Vaccination Law made vaccination compulsory all over what was now the German Empire. In the United States too, municipal and state boards of public health organized smallpox vaccination programmes. Here too popular resistance was common, especially in immigrant communities that felt themselves subjected to prejudiced and excessive attention. Nineteenth-century smallpox vaccination programmes almost everywhere became mired in controversy. In India, despite the commitment of the government of India, disputes arose between officials at central, provincial and local levels. Legislation making vaccination compulsory was even opposed by many officials of the Indian Medical Service on the grounds that it would be impossible to enforce. Brazil, too, had made smallpox vaccination compulsory early in the nineteenth century.

The important point here is that by the time diphtheria sera became available, many countries had established systems for administering and delivering smallpox vaccination. Looking back, we might think that these could easily have been adapted to deliver diphtheria serum. But that was not what happened. To be sure, the incidence of smallpox had been greatly reduced. But because state-mandated vaccination was so unpopular, there was no telling how people would respond to another such programme. Nor were doctors unreservedly enthusiastic, and some saw free vaccination as an encroachment on their professional interests. The proper demarcation between medical practice, concerned with the individual patient, and public health, concerned with the health of the community, was disputed. How did vaccination fit in? Though an intriguing question, this was not a burning issue at the end of the nineteenth century. Vaccination was still associated very much with smallpox and was far from being the mainstay of public health. The emergence of the first diphtheria sera in the course of the 1890s did not at first change anything.

Preventing Diphtheria

At the end of the nineteenth century, diphtheria was a common and widely feared disease. It was largely a children's disease, responsible for thousands of children's deaths. When it became available, in the course of the 1890s, diphtheria antitoxin was used, not to prevent but to treat the disease. Though what exactly the antitoxin did was not known, early experiences were very positive. However it worked, the serum seemed effective. By the mid-1890s children affected by diphtheria were being treated successfully in both Berlin and Paris. Therapeutic use of the serum spread rapidly. In France, the Pasteur Institute established a national network for distributing it without charge, financed by public subscription, by state funds and by exports of serum to other European countries whose governments had ordered it. It was quickly introduced in some London hospitals too, with the result that death rates from diphtheria fell dramatically in the years preceding the outbreak of the First World War. Similar successes were reported from New York, Australia and elsewhere. Nevertheless, despite success in treating the disease, the number of new cases of diphtheria was not falling.

In the 1890s few bacteriologists or physicians thought of using the serum prophylactically, to prevent infection. The idea that vaccination to prevent disease could be extended beyond smallpox only really caught on as a result of experience in the First World War. Insanitary battlefield conditions, a fertile breeding ground for disease, which had claimed many soldiers' lives, stimulated the search for new vaccines, against typhoid in particular. After it was introduced, typhoid vaccine could soon be seen to have saved the lives of thousands of British soldiers. Other countries followed suit in vaccinating their soldiers. As typhoid vaccination was extended, first to nurses working in hospitals, then to missionaries working in the tropics, the idea of preventive vaccination gained terrain. As I pointed out earlier, using diphtheria serum preventively was not simply a logical extension of using it therapeutically. Acceptance of the idea of long-term protection only began to make sense in the light of conceptual breakthroughs then taking place, such as a more subtle understanding of immunity, distinguishing active from passive immunity, and the notion of the uninfected 'carrier'. Empirical developments also played a part: the Schick test for susceptibility, development of toxin–antitoxin mixtures and then of the safer toxoid. These too helped establish the idea of prophylactic vaccination as offering a safe and effective form of protection against a disease. However, as a public health measure, vaccination would be widely judged relative to the measures that had been used previously. Many people thought these measures, which included quarantine and the temporary closure of schools while they were disinfected, were perfectly adequate. What is more, preventive vaccination did not lend itself to the same kind of demonstrations of efficacy as therapeutic vaccination. Doctors and parents alike could witness the recovery of an infected child treated with antitoxin. Whatever the benefits of preventive vaccination, they became visible only gradually, as statistics were collected and analysed. If diphtheria serum was going to be used prophylactically on a large scale, all kinds of new issues would have to be faced. How could adequate and reliable supplies be procured? Would the public health infrastructure enable children to be reached? How would the medical profession react to public health extending beyond sanitation and adopting tools of bacteriology? Physicians in private practice might object to local authorities taking a potentially lucrative practice out of their hands. On the other hand, perhaps many physicians had not been convinced of the value of vaccination in the first place. Nor could anyone be sure how far the unpopularity of smallpox vaccination would affect popular responses to a new mass vaccination campaign.

Nevertheless, influenced by success in saving soldiers from typhoid, in the 1920s and '30s public health officials gradually began to accept the idea of prophylactic diphtheria vaccination. However, differences in geography, resources and access to supplies of serum meant that how exactly it was done differed enormously from place to place. Differing perspectives on the role of the state also played a part. How were responsibilities to be divided between public health authorities and private medical practice, or between central and local government? The consequence of these many influences was that countries and regions differed enormously in the speed with which preventive vaccination against diphtheria began. Parts of Australia, Canada and the United States were at the forefront, starting large-scale preventive vaccination of children in the 1920s.

The Canadian province of Ontario was particularly active. As we saw earlier, John G. Fitzgerald had established an antitoxin laboratory, attached to the University of Toronto, in 1913. As early as 1915 the provincial government had agreed to the free distribution of Fitzgerald's antitoxin – something that the local medical profession firmly supported at the time. Everything was favourable to an effective campaign. There was a cheap and reliable supply of serum, there was enthusiastic leadership from the provincial Board of Health, and doctors did not oppose the measure. In Ontario, immunization became established before resistance to the role of the state in preventive medicine had gathered force. After 1916, Australia also had a cheap and reliable source of antitoxin (and later toxoid) – the Commonwealth Serum Laboratory (CSL). But Australia was vast and thinly populated, its towns and cities separated by huge distances. Moreover, it had only become a single country (the Commonwealth of Australia) in 1901 with the merger of previously independent British colonies. Administrative machinery for a nationwide vaccination programme was not yet established, so that for historical and geographic reasons it was difficult to organize a national vaccination campaign. Even though antitoxin treatment was available, the overall incidence of diphtheria was rising again by the mid-1900s. In 1922, mass vaccination campaigns began in a few communities throughout the country. Vaccination would be offered to children found by Schick testing to be at risk, and it would be voluntary. Toxoid could be obtained from the CSL, but it was a matter for local initiative. In fact most communities did not follow suit for many years, and only with the outbreak of the Second World War did vaccination become routine throughout the country.

In the United States, New York took the lead. The city public health department's laboratory had been producing antitoxin for therapeutic use since as early as 1895, and prophylactic diphtheria vaccination began in 1921. Organizing the mass vaccination of children posed a host of problems. With the cooperation of the city's school system, the public health service (under the leadership of William Park) began mass Schick testing and providing toxin-antitoxin to children – though only those whose parents agreed (an unusual step at the time). However, despite good results it was a struggle. Not only was it proving difficult to reach the pre-school children most at risk, but there was some opposition too. A major publicity effort would be needed if the campaign was to succeed, and the New York health department lacked the resources for this. However, the city's insurance companies, and philanthropic institutions such as the Milbank Memorial Fund, provided the necessary additional funds. The campaign went ahead, and in some communities there were even door-to-door visits to persuade families to ask their doctor for the serum. Newspapers, radio, parades, pageants – all kinds of publicity measures were used in the course of the 1920s. Historian James Colgrove calls it 'a dramatic crusade with eradication of diphtheria as the goal'.[1] Health *education* was becoming established, catalysed by the growth of advertising, and compared to earlier smallpox campaigns this one relied far more on informing and educating and far less on compulsion. Colgrove suggests that this 'marketing' of diphtheria vaccination was viewed with disdain in Britain, 'as alien to British ideas of professional practice'.[2] Not that American physicians in private practice were totally happy about it either, since disagreements were arising regarding whether the vaccination should be offered free by public health centres or obtained (for a fee) from the private physician. The *Journal of the American Medical Association* was against public health centres offering free vaccination.

The British Ministry of Health did little or nothing to initiate mass immunization. Its hesitation was due partly to a reluctance to assume any financial responsibility. But it was also because it was anxious to avoid the risk of antagonizing either GPs (by intruding into fee-paying private practice) or local authorities (by intruding into the realm of local autonomy). If any initiatives were to be taken it was the local medical officers of health who would have to take them. Few did, either because they were not yet convinced of the value of immunization, or because they simply had too much to do already. By this time many were feeling overwhelmed by responsibilities now extending into health services for schools, as well as antenatal and child-welfare clinics. Whatever the explanation, British public health was extremely conservative. Its officers were content to stick to the methods they had used before antitoxin was discovered and, having introduced it, change very slowly once the much safer toxoid became available. The ministry was willing neither to subsidize an immunization campaign nor to give any guidance regarding reliable suppliers (in the absence of a public-sector source of serum supply as in New York or Ontario). Only in the early 1930s did opinion change, and only in 1940, with fears of greater epidemics, did the Ministry of Health provide funding as a temporary wartime emergency measure. It was only in 1941 that a national immunization campaign finally began in England and Wales.

Similar national differences accompanied the start of vaccination against whooping cough (pertussis), from which more than ten thousand American children had died in 1920. In the late 1920s a Danish researcher, Thorvald Madsen, had succeeded in producing a promising vaccine from killed bacilli. Many trials followed, and by the 1930s some doctors in Australia and the USA were starting to offer their patients both therapeutic and prophylactic pertussis vaccination. As with diphtheria serum, many European countries, and Britain in particular, were reluctant to start mass immunization. In Britain the Medical Research Council carried out large-scale clinical trials in the early 1940s. But their results were seen as inconclusive, and leaders of medical opinion were not convinced. New trials were organized, and only after their results had been analysed, in the mid-1950s, did Britain (and other European countries) finally begin mass pertussis vaccination.

Distinctive Traditions and the Introduction of BCG

It is the history of vaccination against tuberculosis, BCG vaccination, that most graphically displays the scepticism towards vaccines that marked some countries' public health policies early in the twentieth century. In the introduction to their classic study of tuberculosis, René and Jean Dubos noted that somewhere between three and five million people died of tuberculosis every year. They were writing in 1952, fully seventy years after Koch's discovery of the bacillus, and thirty years after the first BCG vaccinations.[3] Patterns of tuberculosis mortality in the nineteenth century and the causes of its decline have been among the most contentious of topics in medical and demographic history. Trying to understand why countries responded so very differently to BCG, and why tuberculosis mortality remained so high years after it became available, is scarcely less complex a task. Indeed it is tuberculosis vaccination that best enables us to visualize the vaccination politics of the decades around the Second World War, and to shed some light on the complex of factors that led to widely different responses.

Tuberculosis control did not appear quite the same kind of public health problem as smallpox control or diphtheria control. It tended to show itself only slowly and people could be infected for years without displaying any obvious symptoms. Moreover, symptoms could not always be distinguished from those of other diseases. Many physicians thought that a person's disposition played a major role in whether or not he or she was at risk of becoming 'consumptive', and the important thing, especially for people thought to be of a sensitive disposition, was to be careful. Koch's isolation of the bacterium responsible did not immediately discredit this link between disease and disposition, and still less did it immediately discredit existing ways of treating the condition.

In the course of the nineteenth century, TB sufferers had been subjected to all kinds of treatments. Some of them now sound quite bizarre. Others, including Koch's tuberculin treatment, were soon discredited. On the other hand, the importance of nutrition was recognized in the nineteenth century and is still accepted. Epidemiological studies later demonstrated that a diet rich in meat and milk did help reduce susceptibility to tuberculosis. This helped explain why at times of food scarcity there was often an increased incidence of TB. Rest, and the avoidance of physical exertion, were also prescribed. The recognized association of climate with tuberculosis, and belief in the beneficial effects of clean country, mountain or sea air, gave rise not only to some faddish treatments that at best did no harm, but also to the creation of sanatoria, which offered perhaps the most famous of therapeutic regimes. Many special hospitals for the sequestration of people suffering from pulmonary tuberculosis had been established earlier, but those were different from residential institutions that set out to treat the disease with a healthy open-air regime. A German physician named Herman Brehmer launched the concept when he established what seems to have been the first sanatorium in the Silesian mountains in the 1850s. Despite the fact that many doctors had difficulty accepting that something as simple as fresh air could have therapeutic value, the sanatorium idea grew in popularity. 'Within two decades the concept that tuberculosis could be healed by absolute rest in the open air was accepted all over Europe.'4 The Swiss mountains soon became the resort of choice for those who could afford to go there. A few years later Edward Livingston Trudeau, having read of Brehmer's work, brought the sanatorium to the United States. But tuberculosis was most common among the impoverished inhabitants of urban slums, living in overcrowded conditions that facilitated the spread of infection. Few of those affected were able to take themselves off to the Swiss mountains for a month or two.

The number of deaths from tuberculosis hardly declined in the nineteenth century. Only where public health authorities became convinced of the contagious character of the disease and took action was it brought down. In New York City, for example, and in Prussia, which had the most crowded living conditions of any European country, tuberculosis mortality was reduced after physicians introduced the strict isolation of infected patients. In England and Wales, one investigator found that the decline in tuberculosis mortality was correlated with the extent to which workhouse infirmaries segregated infected patients. A variety of public health measures helped bring down the number of deaths from tuberculosis. They included environmental improvement, such as slum clearance and rehousing to reduce domestic overcrowding; notification by medical practitioners; and clinics and sanatoria that were sometimes paid from public funds. In Britain, local medical officers of health were responsible for coordinating and overseeing these various elements of policy, a role that sometimes brought them into conflict with private medical practitioners who saw their own practice and income threatened.

When British prime minister David Lloyd George introduced the 1911 National Insurance Act, he referred to the implications of tuberculosis for the country. It was killing 75,000 people annually in Great Britain and Ireland, and was responsible for one in three deaths of working-aged males and half of all deaths among young women. He pointed out that Germany, which was investing in the construction of sanatoria, was doing much better. Britain would have to follow suit. If it failed to do so, and did not build the sanatoria, it would fall behind in 'national efficiency'. Three years later the First World War broke out. In the course of the war years, tuberculosis mortality increased enormously, in Britain as in most European countries. Overcrowding, housing shortage, under-nutrition and comorbidity with the 1918 Spanish flu pandemic all are likely to have contributed. After the war, in the 1920s, some countries made BCG vaccination a cornerstone of their efforts at tuberculosis prevention. But once again we see the wide divergence in national policies that we saw also with regard to prophylactic diphtheria vaccination.

At the Hôpital de la Charité in Paris, the vaccine was widely used from the early 1920s onwards. Mixed with milk, it was given orally to newborn babies. In the Scandinavian countries, too, BCG found early champions whose efforts ensured that it was widely used. One of these was Johannes Holm, director of the Danish State Serum Institute (SSI). In Denmark, vaccination with BCG produced by the SSI began in 1927, though large-scale use came only later, at the end of the Second World War. Another important champion was Arvid Wallgren, professor of paediatrics at the University of Gothenburg in Sweden. In 1927 he too began to vaccinate families in which a member was infected. Wallgren played an important role in ensuring the wider introduction of BCG vaccination throughout Sweden. The procedure used in the Scandinavian countries differed from that initially used in France. Whereas the French doctors were administering the vaccine orally, their Scandinavian colleagues injected it under the skin.

German doctors used it too, though only for a while. In Germany BCG vaccination began in 1925, but was halted six years later. In the north German town of Lübeck, 72 children had died within a year of receiving the vaccine. The public outcry was such that BCG vaccination was abandoned, even though a subsequent inquiry found that the accident had been due to contamination of a specific batch of the vaccine. The Lübeck tragedy was of course grist to the mill of the many researchers and physicians who had never believed in BCG. There were many of these sceptics in Britain, where research seemed to cast doubt on both the safety and the effectiveness of BCG vaccination. Even though it was known that the vaccine was being used very effectively in Denmark and Sweden, many in Britain were unwilling to be convinced. After all, they pointed out, there had been no controlled trials in Scandinavia. It was impossible to be sure how much of Danish or Swedish success in controlling tuberculosis was due to the vaccine and how much to these countries' high standard of hygiene and generous provision of hospital beds. Major Greenwood, the eminent London School of Hygiene epidemiologist, dismissed Calmette's data from France as scientifically worthless. Historian Linda Bryder points out that the most statistically convincing trials of BCG, which had been carried out among North American Indians, were viewed as unlikely to be applicable to British people!

Widespread British scepticism towards BCG was not only based on doubts regarding the quality of the evidence for its safety and efficacy. There was a moral, judgemental aspect to it too. Looking at the variation in tuberculosis death rates between the districts of a city, it was clear that they were much higher in poor districts than in better-off ones. Observers of the 1920s were not necessarily inclined to attribute this to differences in the material and environmental conditions under which people lived. Like their Victorian predecessors, medical officers of health were quite likely to see the effect of misguided lifestyle choices, rooted in ignorance and carelessness. Bryder has argued that in attributing the high incidence of tuberculosis mortality to lifestyle choices, tuberculosis specialists wanted to promote a change in lifestyle, and avoid pandering to people's self-indulgences by providing artificial protection.[5] If catching tuberculosis was in large measure a result of ignorant lifestyle choices, then people had to be taught what was good for them and to learn self-control. They had to learn to take responsibility for their health, and to be taught the value of a healthy diet and a lifestyle involving plenty of fresh air and exercise. These were measures that had proved their worth over many years. BCG vaccination would not only give people a false sense of security, it would also reduce the incentive to change their behaviour. Stoking opposition to general tuberculosis vaccination even further was a sense that it threatened doctors' professional and economic interests. Many tuberculosis specialists had appointments as medical superintendents of specialized sanatoria. It is not hard to imagine that they would be predisposed to look sceptically at the evidence for preventive vaccination, which did not seem very strong anyway. The views of tuberculosis specialists in the United States were much the same as those of their British colleagues. In the United States, as in Britain, little use was made of the BCG vaccine. Mass vaccination would interfere with existing practices and might lull people into a false sense of security. Without in any way disputing the seriousness of the condition, British and American tuberculosis specialists largely ignored BCG.

At the outbreak of the Second World War tens of thousands of new cases of tuberculosis were still being diagnosed each year in Britain and there were more than twenty thousand deaths. Just as during the First World War, the death rate from tuberculosis rose during the war years. This was still truer of continental Europe, where rates of tuberculosis shot up as a result of the displacement, homelessness, overcrowding and malnutrition that many countries suffered under Nazi occupation. Neutral Sweden remained at the forefront of anti-tuberculosis vaccination. An emphasis on preventive health fitted well with the extension and intensification of the Swedish welfare state. In 1944 Swedish legislation required that all teachers and schoolchildren who tested negative on the tuberculin test should be offered the vaccine. In Sweden, and at the war's end in Denmark and Norway too, BCG vaccination coverage rose rapidly.

While the war was being fought, British authorities found themselves forced by circumstances to reconsider BCG vaccination. Thanks to the introduction of mass miniature radiography, the newly developed X-ray technique, it had become possible to screen whole populations for early signs of tuberculosis. To start with, mass radiographic screening in Britain focused on army recruits and people working in industries vital to the war effort. This helped stop the spread of infection among them, but it also meant that additional facilities were needed for segregating and treating people found to be infected. And here a problem arose. There was an enormous shortage of nurses to staff the TB sanatoria during and immediately after the war (when radiographic screening was extended to the civilian population). Bryder has shown that women were reluctant to join the profession for fear of becoming infected by the patients they would be nursing. Their fears seem to have been justified. There was a high infection rate among nurses. In 1943 tuberculosis specialists therefore began to urge the Ministry of Health to think again about mass BCG vaccination. Opinion was slowly shifting. At the 1949 Commonwealth and Empire Tuberculosis Conference, a number of delegates argued that vaccination should be introduced in the British colonies. Under conditions prevailing there, where facilities would never equal those available in Britain, mass vaccination would be particularly valuable. Reflecting the slow shift in opinion, in 1949 BCG vaccination was offered to nurses in Britain.

A year later the MRC began a trial among 56,000 schoolchildren. The first results of this trial – suggesting that vaccination offered significant protection – appeared in 1956. But by that time – three years earlier in fact – mass vaccination of children was already under way. The new Labour government had developed its plans for a National Health Service, despite opposition from the organized medical profession. Greater commitment to preventive health fitted with its plans, just as it had with the plans of a Swedish government intent on further developing that country's welfare state.

In Eastern Europe the ravages of resurgent tuberculosis at the war's end were particularly severe. Travelling around Poland in 1946 a Danish Relief Mission found it to be rampant, while local facilities for dealing with it were totally inadequate. Although mass radiography was available in principle, the country's unreliable electricity supplies meant that it was of limited use. In the United States scientists had developed an antibiotic (streptomycin) with which tuberculosis could be treated, but this was in desperately short supply. BCG vaccination seemed the only feasible approach, and in early 1947 a Danish Red Cross team began vaccinating Polish children who tested tuberculin-negative: 46,000 in the first six months of the campaign. Not long thereafter UNICEF, which already had feeding programmes for children in a number of devastated European countries, expressed its willingness to support an extension of what the Danes were doing. At this very same time, planning of the new international health organization, which would soon become the World Health Organization, was under way. Even before the WHO had actually been established, tuberculosis had been recognized as one of the priorities it would have to deal with and an 'Expert Committee on Tuberculosis' was set up in 1947. Johannes Holm, director of the Danish Serum Institute, was appointed chair. Holm, continuing to be based in Copenhagen, would also take charge of UNICEF-supported tuberculosis projects, in which BCG vaccination would be an important – though not the exclusive – approach. His dual role would help to avoid territorial disputes between UNICEF and the new WHO. By early 1948 Norwegian and Swedish relief organizations had agreed to work together with the Danes, and what became known as the 'Joint Enterprise' was established. It would have its headquarters in Copenhagen and apart from work in the field it would also try to standardize testing and vaccination procedures. In 1948 UNICEF's Executive Committee agreed to support the Joint Enterprise with $2 million for its work in Europe – and to provide a further $2 million for vaccination activities in Asia, Africa and Latin America. On 1 July 1948 the Joint Enterprise (later renamed the International Tuberculosis Campaign, or ITC) officially took over the activities that the Danish Red Cross had begun. BCG was supplied by laboratories in Denmark, Sweden, France, India and Mexico, all of which had been approved by the new WHO Committee on Biological Standardization. Because the vaccine was available only as a live vaccine in liquid form, which was sensitive to heat and light and believed to have an effective life of only a few weeks, logistics became vital. The vaccine would have to be moved rapidly from the laboratory to the place at which it was to be used. To start with, it was delivered to field sites by a specially equipped small plane belonging to the Danish Red Cross. As the programme grew, this proved inadequate and in January 1949 the U.S. Air Force loaned the Joint Enterprise a DC3 cargo plane. This was used until, by 1950, commercial flights had become sufficiently reliable and frequent.

The programme was scheduled to last until 30 June 1951, and was thereafter to be integrated into the WHO's regular programme. UNICEF would be responsible for vaccine supplies and individual governments would be responsible for managing the programme within their areas. This was a model that was to be used again when, in 1955, the WHO began its malaria eradication programme.

Over its three years of operation, the ITC carried out programmes of tuberculin testing and BCG vaccination in 22 countries, as well as in Palestinian refugee camps. Thirty million people are said to have been given an initial tuberculin test, and nearly fourteen million were vaccinated. This averages out at more than 27,000 tests and 12,000 vaccinations every day for three years – and this despite the difficulties the campaign ran into in some countries. For example, little work could be done in Italy because the public health authorities there wanted a study rather than a campaign, and there was opposition from the medical profession. In Mexico it seems that testing and vaccination were stopped, restarted and then stopped again, apparently because of a rumour of the vaccine having caused some deaths.

In 1948 the Indian government announced that because TB was assuming epidemic proportions in the newly independent country, it would start its own trial BCG vaccination programme. Indian officials contacted the ITC, and in early 1949 a group of Scandinavian doctors arrived in the country. Their mission was to demonstrate BCG vaccination to Indian doctors in urban centres throughout the country. Though they were originally intended to have remained in India only for six months, they actually stayed until the ITC was absorbed by regular WHO–UNICEF activities in 1951. Thereafter, the Indian authorities took over responsibility for BCG vaccination, and with technical support from the WHO and financial support from UNICEF plans for a mass campaign were laid. It was to be carried out in phases, with seventy million people tested in the first period, and by 1961 the plan was to have tested the whole population below the age of 25 (some 170 million people). The expectation was that vaccinating everybody who tested negative was going to take a full decade of careful work.

For international public health experts the campaign in India represented a considerable challenge. It involved transplanting a way of working that had been developed and implemented in post-war Europe to the very different environment of a poor, hot, densely populated country. Because not everyone was convinced of the safety or the efficacy of BCG, WHO experts wanted campaigns to be as standardized as possible. The mere hint of failure could mean growing opposition to the use of BCG, and this had to be avoided at all costs.

Reconciling local conditions with the pressure from above to work according to a standard protocol proved challenging, and concessions to conditions on the ground soon became unavoidable. Procedures had to be modified from those that were being used in Europe. One tuberculin test to establish if an individual should be vaccinated would suffice, instead of the two that were being used in Europe. Attempts to collect careful statistical data also had to be abandoned. Moreover, while in Europe only qualified medical personnel (doctors and nurses) were allowed to vaccinate, this was simply not feasible in India with its great shortage of medical personnel. Lay vaccinators were recruited to work under the supervision of medical doctors.

Evidence for the efficacy of BCG vaccination in preventing tuberculosis infection was still not totally convincing. The results of trials that had been reported were ambiguous, and certainly did not provide the powerful evidence that would be needed to convince the many sceptics in Britain and the United States. In New York City, W. H. Park (the director of the city department of health's research laboratory, who had been so successful in combatting diphtheria) had begun a trial of BCG in 1927. Park and his colleagues believed that their results, which were totally different from those obtained in the study among American Indians, showed that the vaccine was ineffective. Sceptical researchers in both Britain and the USA continued studying alternative tuberculosis vaccines. For example, with support from the Rockefeller Foundation an alternative inactivated vaccine was tested (without success) in Jamaica in the 1930s. Convinced that the most effective way of dealing with TB was testing, tracing contacts and treatment, leading American specialists continued to oppose mass vaccination with arguments that the British had also used earlier. Vaccination would disrupt existing programmes for identifying and treating people who were infected. If everyone who tested negative on the tuberculin test was given the vaccine then the test would no longer work, and they would be deprived of the best means of tracing sources of infection. In the 1940s streptomycin had become available for treating people with tuberculosis, and American physicians overwhelmingly preferred this option. Even in the 1950s it could plausibly be claimed that there was no really powerful evidence for the effectiveness of the vaccine. It was true that the disease had declined in countries that had introduced it, but one could never be sure how much of the decline was due to the vaccine and how much to the other anti-tuberculosis measures that had also been taken. Moreover, there were a few countries (including Iceland and the Netherlands) that had seen a decline in TB incidence even though little BCG had been used.

American and British experts may have doubted the value of tuberculosis vaccination in their own countries, but they saw that it might be useful in tropical countries where the disease was a far greater threat to health, and where facilities for diagnosing and treating it were limited. For example, tuberculosis was one of the leading causes of death in Brazilian cities such as São Paulo and Rio de Janeiro in the 1930s and '40s, killing more people than typhoid, syphilis, diphtheria or measles. However, Brazil had developed its own BCG vaccine, and from the mid-1940s a vaccination campaign had greatly reduced tuberculosis deaths.

Though evidence was inconclusive, UNICEF and the WHO were committed to BCG vaccination outside Western Europe and North America. Vaccination would have to be an important element in international tuberculosis control. Not the only element, however, and in the WHO (though not in UNICEF) there seem to have been real doubts regarding how far vaccination should be relied upon. But the WHO had little money and no means of developing and implementing any alternative strategy. Mass BCG vaccination was at least relatively cheap and it was feasible. But to convince those who still doubted better evidence for the efficacy of the vaccine was clearly needed. Special studies would have to be set up in order to obtain it, and in the mid-1950s the first steps to obtain such evidence were taken. Somewhat earlier there had been suggestions that the efficacy of the vaccine seemed to vary from place to place. Later reanalysis of data collected from many areas would show scarcely credible variation in the effects of mass vaccination on the incidence of tuberculosis. Some studies found a protective effect of around 80 per cent, while others found none at all. Trying to explain this was an intriguing theoretical problem. But the WHO now faced a major dilemma.

India was the scene of what should have been the ultimate vindi-cation of BCG, but proved to be anything but. Having been proposed some years earlier, in 1968 the largest ever trial of BCG began, in Chingleput District (near to Chennai/Madras). It was conducted by the Indian Council of Medical Research, supported by the WHO and the U.S. Public Health Service. This large trial should establish the value of BCG in tropical conditions definitively and once and for all. The problem at that point was that the most positive assessments had come from countries in which need was lowest. The evidence from poor tropical regions was equivocal at best. The district was chosen because it was known that there was widespread 'low-grade sensitivity' in the population. 'Low-grade sensitivity' had been iden-tified in the 1950s, and had been something of a problem ever since. In certain parts of the world the tuberculin test frequently yielded an ambiguous result: too weak to indicate tuberculosis infection, but clearly something. It was believed to be a consequence of infection with a bacterium related to that causing tuberculosis. There are many species of mycobacteria, some of which are common in soils and not at all pathogenic, and which may have provided some pro-tection against tuberculosis, or may have depressed the working of the vaccine. Inclusion of people with this 'low-grade sensitivity' in a trial would lower the apparent efficacy of the vaccination. Perhaps they were the source of the discrepancy in previous studies? In the new Chingleput trial they were included, as were people testing tuberculin-positive. The methodology of the trial was carefully reviewed by independent experts. In 1977 the first results began to emerge. To the consternation of the Indian medical authorities, and of the WHO, they showed no protective effect whatsoever. Nevertheless, the WHO and the international public health establishment were unwilling to abandon the vaccine, citing a variety of arguments, such as genetic variability of populations, and the fact that the trial had been conducted among adults whereas there was reason to believe the vaccine was more effective in children, but perhaps most important of all, the fact that there was nothing else affordable that could be done. The anti-tuberculosis drugs that had become available were too expensive for widespread use in tropical regions. BCG vaccination was integrated in the high-visibility vaccination programme, the Expanded Programme of Immunization, which the WHO and UNICEF were developing in the early 1970s. Medical opinion swung in favour of the vaccine, despite the evidence from this largest trial. Later studies would confirm that BCG vaccination does prevent severe tuberculosis in children under five years of age and, quite unrelated, offer some protection against leprosy! But TB is resurgent today, especially among HIV-positive people, and there is a search for a new and better vaccine.

Taking Stock: The First Decades

I have tried to construct this account of the start of vaccination around three themes. The first is that instead of regarding vaccines as something unique, as they often seem to be, we should think of them as tools for protecting the health of communities: public health technologies. Doing so allows us to better understand the way in which they were assessed a century ago, before they had become as self-evident as they now are. Thinking about vaccines as tools helps us also to consider effects or uses other than that for which they are ostensibly intended. Tools can be used in all kinds of ways. Everyone knows the example of 'how many uses for a bucket can you think of?' In other words, such a perspective broadens the range of questions we can reasonably ask. It allows us to distinguish between a technology (any technology) and a particular use to which it is being put. I might think the technology of great value but question the way in which some are using it.

Second, acceptance of the value of prophylactic vaccination against diseases other than smallpox was a slow and patchy process. The move from using antitoxin for *treating* diphtheria to using it for *preventing* diphtheria was by no means an obvious or simple one. There were existing ways of containment that many people found perfectly adequate. Successful treatment could easily be observed, whereas the effects of preventive vaccination could only be shown later and with the aid of population-level data. Acceptance of the idea of preventive vaccination depended on better understanding of immunity; on the notion of an asymptomatic carrier; on the development of safer toxoid sera and of Schick testing for susceptibility. Success with typhoid vaccination during the First World War helped convince public health officials that this was a tool that could be more widely used in preventive health. The result was that though antitoxin had been used for treating diphtheria victims since the turn of the century, its large-scale use for preventive purposes dates only from the 1920s. Still many were unconvinced. Even in the 1920s the medical profession was not uniformly enthusiastic regarding bacteriological solutions to problems of health and illness. Some felt that too much was claimed for bacteriology. Wouldn't too exclusive a focus on fighting bacteria mean that constitutional or environmental factors might receive too little attention? Some clinicians, alarmed at the extent to which the laboratory was replacing the bedside as the key site for understanding disease, set about founding a specifically clinical science. Institutions such as the Rockefeller Institute Hospital, which opened in 1914, were emblematic. In 1924 Alfred Cohn, founding editor of the *Journal of Clinical Investigation*, emphasized that while bacteriology was essential to the control of epidemic disease, this was not precisely the principal goal, the essence, of medical practice. As the continuing appeal of sanatorium treatment suggests, and for a host of reasons, many doctors preferred to rely on older approaches, whether to treatment or to disease prevention.

Third, distinctive political and ideological traditions had marked infectious disease control for hundreds of years. The result was that as new sera and vaccines emerged from the laboratory they were deployed in ways that were shaped by these different national traditions (and by international rivalries). How active a role was one government or the other willing to play in fighting diphtheria or any other infectious disease? How legitimate was state intervention perceived to be? What administrative tools did a government – central, regional or municipal – have at its disposal? What was the attitude of the medical profession? Were preventive measures viewed with suspicion, as potentially conflicting with the professional interests of the physician in private practice? Or was the profession supportive of a state role complementary to its own? The start of mass vaccination was marked by concerns regarding the demarcation between central and local government prerogatives and spheres of action, as well as by an unwillingness to intrude into the terrain that the medical profession considered to be that of private practice.

Perhaps it is a little surprising how some of the themes, and the arguments, raised both for and against vaccination in these early years resonate even today. One of the arguments raised against mass tuberculosis vaccination in 1920s Britain invoked 'personal responsibility'. Some people argued that it was a person's own fault if he or she became infected. It was due to lack of self-control and to having made the wrong lifestyle choices. A vaccine that promised protection nonetheless would only reduce the incentive to reflect, and to change behaviour. Nearly a century later this same argument would be used in relation to the human papilloma virus vaccination.

SIX

POLICIES:
VACCINATION AND THE COLD WAR

Between Idiosyncrasy and Ideology

For decades, armed conflict has provided one of the most powerful stimuli to vaccine development. From the First World War onwards, once the value of typhoid vaccination had impressed itself on military commanders, wartime conditions had become a stimulus to their use as well. But the end of hostilities has rarely meant that public health concerns could be allowed to fade into the background. In countries brought to their knees by bombing or occupation, large swathes of the population are left homeless and malnourished as conflict ends. Since these are, of course, the conditions that promote the spread of infectious disease, there is a new health emergency. Today this is an all too familiar scenario. The end of the Second World War left the countries of Central and Eastern Europe in exactly that situation. Tuberculosis was rampant. Since circumstances did not allow for individual case-finding and treatment, the benefits of using BCG to control its spread were clear even to doctors who had previously been sceptical. Though it did not touch the social causes of tuberculosis, BCG vaccination came to seem a useful technological fix under prevailing circumstances. In Britain too, it was the circumstances of the time that led to a reappraisal. The years immediately following the end of the war saw British scepticism trumped first by shortage and then by new political commitment to establishing a welfare state. So it may seem that the differences in countries' recourse to vaccination in the 1920s and '30s, rooted in differing political ideologies and administrative and professional practices, would have begun to fade by the 1950s.

However, the years following the end of the Second World War saw the industrialized world increasingly polarized. As regards official ideologies, administrative and political practices, the organization of production, social services and freedom of expression, the centrally planned economies of Eastern and Central Europe differed from the Western free-market economies in these and many other respects. Since predominant views regarding public health constituted one such respect, we can also imagine a new logic imposing itself in the vaccine field. So far as the deployment of vaccines is concerned, perhaps what post-war decades show is not so much the fading of idiosyncrasy as vaccines' partial subordination to a new order. So the question now is: how did these new political configurations affect the utilization of vaccines as public health technologies? Not their development. In the 1950s and '60s both sides were united in their shared faith in science as the basis of progress. And as the history of Albert Sabin's polio vaccine shows, scientists found ways of circumventing political barriers to the exchange of scientific information. Public health policies, however, were a different matter. As historian Dora Vargha puts it, 'Although the development of the live [polio] vaccine was the result of intensive cooperation across the Iron Curtain, its implementation followed Cold War fault lines.'[1] East and West had different visions of how public health should develop, both at home and in the newly independent countries of the developing world in which, by the 1950s, they were competing for influence. Politicians on both sides of the ideological divide felt that noteworthy success in controlling epidemic disease, in preventing unnecessary loss of life, would reflect well on their political system.

Cold War Rhetoric

In international arenas, with representatives of both blocs present, Cold War tensions were often quite explicit. Discussions of international public health were no exception. In the spring of 1946, eighteen experts met in Paris to plan a successor to the Health Organization of the pre-war League of Nations (of which the USA had never been a member and from which the Soviet Union had actually been expelled). At a large international gathering of government representatives in New York a few months later their proposals for a new organization were debated. At the conclusion of this meeting, 61 states signed the constitution of what, in April 1948, would become the World Health Organization (WHO). The new organization would have its headquarters in Geneva; a 'parliament', the World Health Assembly (WHA), which would meet annually to fix the organization's budget and the broad lines of its activities; and regional offices in the various continents. To start with, the fledgling WHO continued the work of its predecessor organization, but it soon developed its own list of priorities. The topics to which it attached the highest importance have a familiar ring to them even now – malaria, maternal and child health, and tuberculosis. But in no time at all the new political cleavages were starting to become visible. So much so that the organization was soon shaken to its foundations. Although the Soviet Union and its allies had joined the WHO when it was founded, within a few months they had left (though the WHO's constitution didn't allow for actual resignation). Eastern bloc countries claimed that the organization was not doing what they expected of it, that its administrative costs were too high, and that it was dominated by the USA.

The organization's principal activity in the 1950s – the worldwide anti-malaria campaign launched in 1955 – was indeed an initiative of the United States. It is also true that within two or three years this programme had become the most extensive of all WHO activities, financed from a special fund and operating in over fifty countries. There had previously been a major malaria eradication effort in the Americas, and the WHO's Brazilian director general, a parasitologist named Marcelino Candau, was attracted to the idea of a global campaign. President Eisenhower was persuaded that U.S. support for such an initiative could be a useful antidote to growing Communist influence in Africa and Asia. Within two years the U.S. was bearing the brunt of what was becoming a vast international project, costing millions of dollars and involving a staff of hundreds. At the same time, the focus of the programme was gradually shifting from simply controlling malaria to the much more ambitious goal of totally eradicating it. No large-scale vaccination was involved, since there was no malaria vaccine. Rather, the campaign involved attacking the mosquitoes through clearing away their swampy breeding grounds, spraying houses with DDT and providing villagers with mosquito nets for protection while asleep. Optimists suggested that malaria would be eradicated within a few years.

Then, in 1957, the Soviet Union and its allies rejoined the WHO and began to urge reconsideration of the organization's priorities.

The Soviet delegation to the 1958 World Health Assembly (WHA) was led by Victor Zhdanov, a virologist and deputy minister of health of the USSR. Zhdanov proposed to the WHA that the organization commit itself to a *smallpox* eradication campaign. His country had succeeded in stopping smallpox transmission years before, despite the country's poor health infrastructure. Nevertheless, because the disease was constantly being imported by travellers arriving at the borders, the country could not discontinue its costly vaccination programme. Zhdanov argued that transmission would be halted if 80 per cent of the population was vaccinated, and if this could be accomplished on a global scale vaccination could cease everywhere.

Although the assembly accepted Zhdanov's proposal, the director general was unenthusiastic. The organization was still committed to malaria eradication, and this commitment was backed by the United States, the WHO's largest contributor. Not only was Candau personally sceptical as to the feasibility of smallpox eradication, but he was also reluctant to see resources diverted from the attack on malaria. Thus although in 1958 smallpox eradication officially became a WHO priority, virtually no resources were devoted to it. Each year thereafter the Soviet delegate expressed his frustration at the lack of progress.

By the early 1960s there was mounting evidence that the malaria campaign was going to fail. In the U.S. there were accusations that funds were being misused, and domestic political support was crumbling. Internationally, support for the programme was giving way to a sense that it would have to be abandoned. This left the United States government, which had been the eradication programme's major supporter, in something of a dilemma. In 1965 the first American combat troops arrived in Vietnam. In much of the developing world the country's reputation was being seriously damaged by its military involvement in Indochina. A high-profile engagement in the field of health should help mitigate the diplomatic damage, but malaria eradication was failing and could no longer serve that purpose. The American government was anxious to associate itself with an alternative humanitarian endeavour.

At the 1965 assembly the United States delegation therefore switched its attention to smallpox. Allying itself with the USSR, the U.S. delegation now argued for a concerted attack on that disease. The director general was asked to draw up a specific plan, to be presented to the following year's assembly. When it was, it was hotly debated, not least because it would require a substantial increase in the WHO budget. Many delegates were surprised when the assembly accepted the plan, though by a very small margin. Who was going to be put in charge of this new 'intensified' smallpox eradication programme? The delegation of the Soviet Union thought it should be a Russian, since not only had the programme been their idea, but also they were the only country that could produce the vaccine on a large enough scale. Still sceptical, the director general thought it should be an American. He asked the U.S. surgeon general to nominate someone. Donald Henderson, chief of the surveillance section at the CDC, was selected to go to Geneva to run the programme and the WHO's new Smallpox Eradication Unit.

Cold War Practice: Polio Vaccination

Each bloc was keen to take every opportunity of extolling its technological and moral superiority to the other. But the resulting rhetorical positioning which took place in international fora such as the World Health Assembly tells us little about actual public health practice or about changes in the ways vaccines were being used. An example, to be set against the examples of diphtheria and tuberculosis discussed in the previous chapter, can throw light on changes in vaccine politics. Polio vaccines, becoming available from the mid-1950s, offer such an example. What can we learn from their introduction and use? Did national idiosyncrasies fade still further, or were they rather displaced, or overlaid, by ideological polarization?

Although there had been outbreaks of polio in the late nineteenth century, polio victims had mostly been children aged between about six months and four years of age. In young children the disease tended to manifest itself in flu-like symptoms and cases of paralysis were rare. In the twentieth century, as the first large-scale epidemics were documented, it became clear that both the scale and the severity of polio infections had changed dramatically. The United States was particularly affected, and an epidemic that struck New York in 1916 caused widespread panic. Thousands of people fled the city, theatres and cinemas closed, and children were told to avoid public places and above all not to drink from water fountains. In the years around the First World War, public health authorities tended to approach polio epidemics in the same way, using the same tools that had been used with epidemics of other infectious diseases. It was taken for granted that the disease was the result of poor hygiene, lack of sanitary facilities, poverty. The response, reflecting established approaches to the control of epidemics, thus involved slum clearance and cleaning, restrictions on mobility, and sometimes the quarantining of poor neighbourhoods.[2] It didn't help. The epidemics kept on returning, and every summer one or other region of the United States was struck. There was a particularly serious epidemic in 1949, with 2,720 deaths from the disease in the United States and 42,173 cases. In the UK, though numbers were far smaller, there too rates of infection peaked in the immediate post-war years. In 1947 there were nearly eight thousand cases in England and Wales, or ten times the number recorded a year earlier. It was unclear why this had happened. Some thought it was a result of the unusually dry summer of 1947. Others blamed food rationing and poor nutrition. Yet others speculated that returning soldiers had brought a new and more virulent strain back with them. By the 1950s polio had become a major public health problem in Britain.

By that time researchers in the United States had made considerable progress in understanding the disease. In the 1920s it had already become clear that spread of infection could not be controlled with the old methods, since middle-class neighbourhoods, not poor ones, were most severely affected. By the 1940s the reasons for this were better understood, thanks to epidemiological studies carried out in different regions of the world. Babies rapidly acquired passive immunity from their mothers. As this waned, children in less hygienic environments acquired some natural immunity from their environment. Better hygiene meant that infants and young children had fewer opportunities to encounter and develop immunity to polio. Exposure to polio virus was therefore delayed until late childhood or adult life, when it was more likely to take the paralytic form.

New treatments were developed in the 1920s and '30s, including a serum that was thought to reduce the risk of infection leading to paralysis. However, at this time polio was rarely diagnosed before paralysis appeared and by that time the serum would no longer help. In the 1930s affected children were commonly immobilized during the acute and convalescent phases of the disease: strapped to boards sometimes for months at a time, they would have to be carried around by their parents. Then came Sister Elizabeth Kenny, an Australian nurse, who became a famous critic of the immobilization practice. Her alternative method, which became popular in the 1940s, involved heating and re-educating affected muscles with physiotherapy. The most serious cases were those in which the muscles that control breathing or swallowing became paralysed. The artificial breathing device known as the 'iron lung' saved the lives of many severely afflicted patients who would otherwise have died. Unfortunately the first iron lungs were extremely expensive. In the 1930s, an iron lung cost about $1,500 – about the same price as the average home. By the end of the 1940s they had become more common and hospital wards were filled with them. It saved lives, but patients remained encased in the metal chambers for months or years, and sometimes for life. Even with an iron lung the fatality rate for patients with the most serious form of polio was very high. Their occupants were generally adults, including pregnant women, a few of whom even gave birth while inside one.

The years following the Second World War saw more and more regions (not only North America, Australia and Europe but also South and Central America, the Middle East, the Soviet Union and Asia) struck at intervals by increasingly severe epidemics. At this time a new serum containing antibodies against polio was prepared from the blood of survivors. This serum, it was thought, would prevent the spread of polio and reduce the severity of disease. It did seem to be about 80 per cent effective in preventing the development of paralytic poliomyelitis. Unfortunately, however, the immunity it provided seemed to last only for about five weeks, so that a new dose would be required each time an epidemic broke out. Moreover, though the antibody serum was widely used in the United States, producing it was an expensive and time-consuming process.

This was the context in which Salk's polio vaccine made its appearance. Within two hours of the trial results being announced, in 1955, the vaccine was licensed for use in the United States. Preparations for vaccinating five million American children began immediately. There was no trace of the scepticism that continued to mark American doctors' attitude to tuberculosis vaccination with BCG.

Polio had a visibility in the United States unmatched anywhere else. It was here, as we saw earlier, that the bulk of the research on polio was being conducted. But with the vaccine's licensing, European countries too began to consider the desirability of polio vaccination. Their initial responses were as different from one another as responses to the development of new vaccines had been in the past. The varied responses of the different European countries did not reflect differences in the numbers of inhabitants killed or paralysed by polio over the years. Authorities were goaded into action less by reflection on historical data than by public anxieties. It was frequently a *recent* epidemic, a crisis fresh in people's minds and memories, that provided the stimulus. Danish authorities acted rapidly because the country had been shaken by an epidemic of unprecedented severity in 1952. The Dutch were initially more hesitant, taking no action until 1956, when the Netherlands too was struck by a serious epidemic. Then the government decided to import vaccine and offer free vaccination to all children up to fourteen years of age. The epidemic also led the Dutch government to try to make vaccination programmes more efficient by integrating what had previously been local responsibilities into a more centralized National Immunization Programme.

The British authorities reacted more enthusiastically than their Dutch counterparts to start with, but then hesitated when the Cutter incident became known. There was a sense that it might be better not to import vaccine from the U.S., and that locally produced vaccine should be used in a trial programme. Vaccine would be offered to children aged between two and nine, who would have to be registered in advance. However, this half-hearted campaign, which took place in 1956, led to the vaccination of only 3 per cent of the group of children at which it was aimed. But professional opinion was changing, and public pressure was building up. The result was that in 1958 the British government agreed that all children under fifteen would be vaccinated. The preference was still for domestically produced vaccine, which should include a less aggressive strain than the one Salk had used in his vaccine. Despite the fact that it would cost more than importing vaccine from North America, the sense that it would be safer was felt to justify the extra cost. However, discussions with manufacturers showed that the quantity of vaccine being produced in the UK was insufficient for a national programme. Vaccine would have to be imported, though imported vaccine would be subjected to additional testing in Britain. Parents would also have the right to refuse to allow their children to be vaccinated with imported vaccine. Though the national programme gathered pace only slowly, once sufficient quantities of vaccine were available it proceeded smoothly under the auspices of the National Health Service.

Faced with an epidemic, or memories of a recent epidemic, European politicians were under pressure to respond. But their ability to mount an effective response, to take advantage of the new vaccines, depended on their influence over health services, and this in turn depended on the role of the state in their finance and organization. Central control and finance made it much easier to mount an effective mass vaccination programme. Thus Britain had its National Health Service, and by the late 1950s the Netherlands had a centrally organized National Immunization Programme. With a very weak central health service administration the German Federal Republic (West Germany) was at the other extreme, at least as far as Europe was concerned. It had no federal ministry of health, but only a department within the Ministry of the Interior. Most public health issues, including vaccination, were the responsibility of the individual states, or *Länder*. Each one, separately, had to license vaccines, to obtain them, to issue laws or decrees on how to deal with vaccination. As a result polio vaccination began unevenly: free in some places and only on payment in others. Making matters more complicated still was the fact that many leading West German health officials and scientists still mistrusted u.s. vaccine research. The result was a slow, patchy start to polio vaccination, with campaigns even occasionally grinding to a halt in some areas.

Cold War attitudes to American technology notwithstanding, East European countries responded as rapidly as those of Western Europe. Czechoslovakia and Poland were soon able to produce their own inactivated vaccine and they started using it in 1957, the same year as the Dutch. Hungary was in a different situation when it too was struck by a major polio epidemic in 1957. The country was still shaking from a revolution forcibly put down by Russian tanks just months earlier. Although plans for producing Salk vaccine had been laid, and in 1956 Hungarian experts had gone to the Danish Serum Institute to study the process, political and social disruption meant that production could only start in 1959. In the meantime something had to be done, and IPV was imported from Canada. However, both import of Salk vaccine, and plans for producing it domestically, were soon overturned.

While the Salk vaccine was being introduced in Europe, Albert Sabin's attenuated vaccine was still being tested. In early 1956 a group of senior Soviet virologists travelled to the USA to learn about polio vaccine production, visiting both Salk's and Sabin's laboratories. With the approval of the State Department and the FBI, Sabin, who was, of course, of Russian birth, established a collaboration with Chumakov's laboratory in Leningrad (now St Petersburg). It was through this collaboration that Sabin was able to arrange a large-scale test of his vaccine: not in the USA, as Salk's had been, but in the USSR (and also, on a smaller scale, in some of its allies). When the Sabin vaccine was licensed in the United States it was almost immediately adopted in place of the Salk vaccine, reflecting a widespread professional consensus that it would be quicker-acting and more effective. Manufacturers followed suit. So did most national governments, though not those of the Netherlands or of the Nordic countries. In Britain the vaccination programme using the Salk vaccine seemed to be working well and millions of people had been vaccinated. Experts thought that the Sabin vaccine should be kept in hand, though, and should be reserved for an emergency. In September 1961 there was a serious outbreak in the city of Hull, and the supply of OPV, kept for just such an emergency, was dispatched to the city. The epidemic was soon brought under control. This success triggered rethinking on the part of the government's health advisers, and, by early 1962, plans were being made for a switch to vaccination using the Sabin vaccine. For the communist states of Central and Eastern Europe, an additional factor played a role in the decision to switch from the Salk to the Sabin vaccine. It was not simply that Sabin's OPV was favoured by professional opinion. Sabin's vaccine looked ideologically better, thanks to its roots on 'their' side of the Iron Curtain.

In divided Germany, Cold War rivalries played out particularly visibly. The Federal Republic, and more specifically the western half of Berlin (which had a special administrative status), developed policies with one eye on what the East Germans were doing. East Germany (the German Democratic Republic) began polio vaccine using the Sabin vaccine in April 1960 and within a year had vaccinated almost the whole population. The Federal Republic, by contrast, had only succeeded in vaccinating its population very patchily with IPV. The consequences of such successes and failures extended beyond matters of public health or lives saved. They reflected well or badly on the ideological systems from which they emerged. So the implications of West Germany clearly lagging behind the East went far beyond concern with polio as a public health issue. Ideological competition between the two German states was one factor that goaded the West German authorities into action. Another was international pressure, because at international conferences the Federal Republic's poor polio vaccination coverage became a matter of growing embarrassment for the country's delegates. Initiatives were taken that only a few years earlier had been politically inconceivable. The West German *Länder*, which had acted so slowly and disjointedly in starting IPV vaccination, now jostled with each other to be the fastest and the most efficient in introducing free OPV vaccination. The programme was an immediate success; 23 million people were vaccinated in 1962, and numbers of cases of polio declined rapidly. By June 1960 over fifty million people had been given the Sabin vaccine worldwide. They lived in the United States, Canada, Mexico, China, the Soviet Union, Czechoslovakia, the United Kingdom and other European countries. (A few million more, mainly in Africa and Latin America, had been given rival live vaccines developed by Koprowski and by Cox.)

Collaboration in Practice

By the 1960s, smallpox had more or less disappeared from the United States and from Europe. However, it was still rampant in parts of Latin America, in Africa and above all in Asia. Since the liquid vaccine that had been used in Western Europe could not withstand the high temperatures of tropical countries for more than a day or two, its use in such countries would be limited. However, some years before, Leslie Collier, a virologist working at the Lister Institute of Preventive Medicine in London, had developed a method for large-scale production of a freeze-dried vaccine that could be reconstituted by mixing it with saline solution. This could survive high temperatures for about a month, making it suited to use in hot countries. The USSR had established facilities for producing freeze-dried smallpox vaccine on a large scale, and there were more limited production facilities in a few other countries. The availability of this thermally stable vaccine, combined with Henderson's leadership and the WHO's new strategy of 'surveillance and containment' (which called for weekly reports of outbreaks and the dispatch of special containment teams to deal with them), were transforming the attack on smallpox. Freeze-dried vaccine was supplied to countries in which smallpox was endemic and in West and Central Africa there was rapid progress. With material and personnel support from the USA, between January 1967 and December 1969 100 million people were vaccinated against smallpox in the twenty-country region. In May 1970 the last cases were reported there.

However, implementation of the campaign was not as effective everywhere, and progress was patchy. Something like 100,000 new cases of smallpox were still being reported each year, 30–40,000 of them in India. Some rethinking was required if smallpox was really going to be wholly and finally eradicated. Previous estimates had been over-optimistic. It had been assumed that if 80 per cent of people in a community were vaccinated, transmission would be halted. Now it was starting to seem that this would not be enough. In India, smallpox had been found to persist in some areas despite vaccination rates of 80 per cent or more. The goal would have to be to vaccinate everybody: 100 per cent of the population.

Powerful backing at the global level, even when it came from both superpowers, was no guarantee of success. Other stumbling blocks also lay in wait for the global programme, including regional conflicts and nationalist resistance to interventions imposed from outside. These problems were particularly acute in the Indian subcontinent, where a 1971 war saw Bangladesh break loose from Pakistan. Hundreds of thousands were killed, and many more, perhaps millions, fled to neighbouring India. Regionalism, heightened nationalist sentiments, and ethnic and religious divisions all meant that the WHO-led programme did not have an easy passage in the region. By 1973 there were still tens of thousands of new cases of smallpox annually. The Indian subcontinent was singled out for concentrated international attention, and large numbers of foreign (mainly American) physician–epidemiologists were flown into the region. The strategy then adopted was that everyone in a village in which a case of smallpox had been identified was to be vaccinated.

Known as the 'ring-fence' strategy, this meant that whether an individual had been vaccinated earlier and was already immune was of no consequence. Nor was consent requested, and where necessary people who objected were vaccinated by force.

The smallpox eradication programme was an international initiative in which the two superpowers could collaborate. It was not strategically important enough to much concern the top levels of political leadership. There was a division of labour, with the u.s. supplying most of the money and skilled personnel, and the ussr most of the vaccine. The medical and scientific people centrally involved, experts such as Henderson and Venediktov, had no difficulty in working together towards an objective such as this.

Alternative Visions

Despite the credit it could take from having put smallpox eradication on the political agenda, the ussr had no deep-rooted commitment to disease eradication. In most international gatherings, Soviet delegations emphasized a vision for the future of public health with a quite different focus. In 1970 Venediktov, who led the Soviet delegation to the World Health Assembly, told fellow delegates that the ussr wished to introduce a resolution on 'the scientific or rational principles upon which the development of a national public health system should be based'.[3] Socrates Litsios, who worked for the who at the time, recalls an intense debate on two elements of the draft resolution: the role of the state, and charges for healthcare. The Soviet delegation argued that the state should be fully responsible for the provision of health services, and that this should be based on a national plan. Because the u.s. delegation objected to this a compromise had to be found. The Soviet delegation's initial formulation had also demanded provision of the 'highest possible level of skilled, universally available medical care, free of charge'. This, of course, hardly chimed with a healthcare system based almost exclusively on fee-paying and private practice, as in the United States. Again a compromise had to be found, so that the final resolution, adopted by the assembly, referred to the 'highest possible level of skilled universally available preventive and curative medical care, without financial or other impediments'.

Delegations from the Soviet Union and its allies were not alone in arguing that public health around the world was best served by prioritizing the extension of basic healthcare. Many of the WHO's own staff held similar views. It was difficult to see how a commitment to extending and improving primary healthcare could be reconciled with a single-minded focus on eradication of a specific disease, whether it was malaria, smallpox or anything else. Many WHO officials, especially those working in the regional offices, believed that the key priority had to be enhancing countries' capacity to deliver basic health services to their people. From this perspective, a programme like smallpox eradication, devouring vast resources, was a regrettable step in the wrong direction. Indeed, not long after the WHA vote that launched the 'intensified' eradication programme, two of the organization's top officials wrote to regional offices advising them to consider taking funds from the eradication programme in order to strengthen basic health services in their region. After all, the argument went, the eradication programme could only succeed if such services had been established and were functioning adequately.

The 1970s were marked by continuing debate regarding whether the priority in international health should be to extend and improve basic health services or to target specific diseases. This antagonism between supporters of what became known respectively as 'horizontal' and 'vertical' approaches would have major implications for discussion of how future immunization programmes should be organized. Although it had roots in Cold War politics, the opposition between these alternative visions was not simply an expression of Cold War antagonisms. A strong commitment to one view or the other could have its roots in professional experience rather than in political ideology. In 1973 Halfdan Mahler, a Danish tropical diseases specialist who had been adviser to the Indian tuberculosis control programme, became the WHO's third director general. Mahler was very much in favour of resources going to basic health services rather than to prestige projects. In this he agreed with the proposal coming from the USSR and its allies. However, he disagreed with them in one important respect. Mahler wanted initiatives to come from the bottom up, rather than following from a central plan, as in Soviet proposals. While the smallpox campaign was slowly moving along, the WHO was developing a vision for the future of public health that fitted with Mahler's values and commitments.

In 1975 the WHO and UNICEF jointly produced a report entitled 'Alternative Approaches to Meeting Basic Health Needs in Developing Countries'. This report, which was profoundly to influence WHO thinking in the following years, was critical of 'vertical' programmes focused on specific diseases while ignoring the poverty, ignorance and squalor that were the real sources of ill health in developing countries. Drawing on 'Alternative Approaches', at the 1976 Health Assembly Mahler proposed the goal of 'health for all by the year 2000'.

Mahler's commitment helped pave the way for a conference on primary healthcare that took place in Alma Ata, Kazakhstan, in September 1978. The Declaration of Alma Ata, affirmed by the conference, emphasized the importance of health for socio-economic development. It criticized reliance on sophisticated medical technologies that would never be available to everyone. Primary healthcare, which where necessary made use of lay health personnel, encouraged community participation, and was integrated with other aspects of socio-economic development, should form the cornerstone of public health. The 1979 World Health Assembly endorsed the declaration, and agreed that primary healthcare was the key to attaining an acceptable level of health for all.

It did not take long for dissenting voices, mostly American, to make themselves heard. In 1979, Julia Walsh and the Rockefeller Foundation's Kenneth Warren, writing in the *New England Journal of Medicine*, argued that, however laudable, the Alma Ata declaration was unrealistic.[4] The costs of providing clean water, nutritional supplements and even the most basic primary healthcare for the world's population could never be met. Walsh and Warren introduced the concept of 'selective primary healthcare'. Attention and resources should be focused on the most serious diseases, and specifically on those for which simple and effective technologies of prevention or control were available. On this basis they classified diseases into 'high', 'medium' and 'low' priorities. The 'high' category included diarrhoeal diseases, measles, whooping cough, malaria and neonatal tetanus; the 'medium' category included polio, respiratory infections, tuberculosis and hookworm; while in the 'low' category were leprosy, diphtheria and Leishmaniasis. Selective primary healthcare should then take as its priority control of the diseases they had ranked most highly, but only in so far as proven technologies were available. Priority should be given to providing tetanus toxoid for pregnant women, to the encouragement of long-term breastfeeding, to providing chloroquine for young children in malaria-infested areas, to oral rehydration packets, and to universal vaccination using DPT and measles vaccine.

New Configurations: Measles Vaccination

In the early 1970s smallpox vaccination was discontinued in the United States and in most of Western Europe. But before that happened, new vaccines were already being introduced. As with the polio vaccines a few years previously, they were being introduced in ways that still reflected different histories, administrative practices and ideological commitments.

In nineteenth-century Britain measles had taken the lives of between 10 and 20 per cent of children who became infected. After the Second World War, antibiotics had made it possible drastically to reduce deaths from measles, and in Britain they had fallen from more than three hundred in 1949 to less than a hundred ten years later. They were still falling in the early 1960s when the first measles vaccines were licensed in the United States. The Federal United States government had only recently become involved with immunization, with 1962 legislation designed to stimulate the immunization of all children against polio, diphtheria, whooping cough and tetanus. But since most immunizations were done by doctors in private practice, and since large swathes of uninsured people never saw a doctor, a result had been that infectious diseases were becoming increasingly concentrated among the urban poor. In the context of the Kennedy and the Johnson administrations' commitment to poverty reduction and the extension of social welfare provision – Johnson launched his Great Society programme in 1964 – this shocking discovery demanded a response. The 1962 legislation was renewed and measles immunization was added. By 1966 the reported incidence of measles had been reduced by about half and was still falling. Nevertheless, public health officials at the CDC lobbied for a campaign aiming at complete elimination of measles from the United States. 'To those who ask me "Why do you wish to eradicate measles?"' wrote Alexander Langmuir, the CDC's chief epidemiologist at the time, 'I reply with the same answer that Hillary used when asked why he wished to climb Mt. Everest. He said: "Because it is there." To this may be added . . . and it can be done.'[5]

Langmuir was expressing a faith in the limitless possibilities of (American) science that was characteristic of the time. Faith in science had never been as boundless as it was in the early 1960s, and would never be so again. But healthcare involves more than science alone, and more than the sophisticated tools that science can provide. Even if vaccination were going to be available to all, including to poor people unable to pay, parents would still have to be convinced it was in their child's interest. Merck, which was supplying the measles vaccine, took on this task and launched a huge advertising campaign designed to 'rebrand' measles as a truly threatening disease. But despite this, and despite backing from President Johnson, the anti-measles campaign was not a total success. Though not all parents were convinced that they should have their children vaccinated against measles, this was only part of the explanation. Congressional support – and hence the campaign's budget – fluctuated wildly from year to year. The result was that though the number of cases of measles declined, the elimination objective remained out of reach.

Langmuir's justification for an all-out attack on measles, 'because it can be done', did not resonate with the more cautious views of European public health officials. When the first measles vaccines became available, the response in Britain was as cautious as it had been with most previous vaccines. Not all British experts were convinced of the wisdom of mass measles vaccination. Those who were stressed the prevalence of the disease. In a typical year there would be something like 35,000 children with serious complications from measles, of whom about six thousand would need to spend some days in hospital. This wasn't a large proportion of the nation's children, but it did represent a significant burden to parents and to the health service. On the other hand, since British parents tended to see a measles episode as an inevitable aspect of childhood, there was a real possibility they wouldn't think their child needed to be vaccinated against it. If that happened there was the risk that parents would start to question the vaccination programme more generally. The British government's view was that, in considering the introduction of a new vaccine, maintaining popular confidence in the immunization programme as a whole had to be a priority.

Moreover, little was as yet known regarding the duration of the immunity conferred by measles vaccine. If it proved to be no more than a few years, people would become vulnerable to infection at a later age. And if that happened, if measles epidemics hit adults rather than children, the complications were potentially much more serious. Nor was it clear which vaccine should be used or according to what schedule. So far as British policymakers were concerned a number of questions would have to be answered before any decisions could be taken. This was why the Medical Research Council began a study of measles vaccination in 1964. Only when its results were available, in 1967, were decisions taken. The Joint Committee on Vaccination and Immunisation, the British government's principal expert advisory body on vaccination policy, recommended that all children aged one year and older who had not had measles and had not been vaccinated should be given live attenuated measles vaccine. The recommendation was accepted, and in 1968 mass vaccination began in Britain, even though it was still unclear for how many years protection would last.

Other Western European countries, perhaps especially those with well-organized welfare systems and highly efficient vaccination programmes, were even more hesitant. In Sweden mass measles vaccination began in 1971 and in the Netherlands only in 1976. Their hesitancies reflect caution, and concern with the questions that would have to be answered before decisions could responsibly be taken. They also reflect a concern, which was shared with Britain, about the implications for the national immunization programme as a whole. There was a fear that introducing a vaccine few parents wanted could undermine popular confidence in immunization programmes more generally: programmes that were working very well.

In Eastern and Central European countries there were no such concerns. Their authoritarian systems of government and state healthcare provision meant that what parents may have wanted was less important. People did not have to be persuaded and there was no need for American-style advertising campaigns. Measles vaccination started rapidly. In what is now Croatia (and was then the Croatian Republic of Yugoslavia), the internationally respected Zagreb vaccine institute was soon able to provide the country with a ready supply of measles vaccine. Vaccination began there in 1964, and in 1968 a single dose was made mandatory for all children. Hungary began measles vaccination in 1969, using a vaccine produced in the Soviet Union. In mass campaigns a single dose of the vaccine was given to children aged 9–27 months. Following a large epidemic in 1973-4, primarily among unvaccinated six- to nine-year-olds, in 1974 the mass campaigns were discontinued. Thereafter the vaccine was integrated into routine child healthcare, given to babies at the age of ten months (fourteen months from 1978). Coverage rates of well over 90 per cent were soon achieved.

Though they started rather differently, measles vaccination programmes in North America and Europe were all successful. Numbers of cases of measles fell dramatically, and thanks to the availability of antibiotics few children died even if they did catch measles. But in the rest of the world, in Africa, Asia and parts of Latin America, measles was as serious in the 1960s as it had been in Europe at the beginning of the century. There were reports from some African countries of 10–20 per cent case fatality. That means that of children diagnosed as having measles 10–20 per cent died: comparable with Britain in the nineteenth century (and now believed to be due to an immune system depressed by the effects of malnutrition). There were few accurate mortality and morbidity statistics at this time, and epidemiological data for much of the world were patchy and unreliable. But there were estimates: striking enough to have political impact. The death rate from measles in developing countries was estimated to be 56 times greater than in developed countries. For some other diseases against which vaccines were available, the difference was even greater: for diphtheria one hundred times greater, and for whooping cough three hundred times greater. If vaccination against these diseases could be extended to the developing world, millions of children's lives could be saved.

Global Action: Acting and Justifying

The smallpox campaign was working well in Africa. Experts in international health were starting to wonder whether it provided a blueprint on which other vaccination programmes might be modelled. In late 1973 the WHO set up an internal working group to flesh out the idea. Introducing a meeting of the working group, the assistant director general explained what the Secretariat had in mind.

Communicable diseases were by far the most important public health problems in the developing areas of the world, accounting for more than half of the ten principal causes of death. What is more, the dramatic effects of many of these killer diseases could be greatly reduced if children were vaccinated. Experience in the northern hemisphere showed that smallpox, diphtheria, pertussis, tetanus, poliomyelitis and measles, and to some extent tuberculosis and typhoid fever, could be virtually eliminated. Anyone who reads the report of this consultation meeting will soon see that it had been drafted in full awareness of the ideological cleavage in the international public health field. On the one hand, inspiration is drawn from the WHO's tuberculosis and smallpox campaigns, 'the success of these programmes makes mandatory an attempt to extend the value of immunization across a wider spectrum of diseases', and '[t]he challenge is to find ways to maximize the benefits of immunization by administering as many effective antigens as possible to as many children as possible, as soon after birth as is consonant with immunological, logistical and economical constraints.' But the new director general's commitment to strengthening primary healthcare also shines through: 'Each country will need to develop a programme suitable to its conditions.' For example,

> the delivery component . . . should take into consideration local conditions, e.g. harvesting season, market days etc. The programmes must be organized in such a way as to accommodate different needs of different population groups in different localities (for example migrant population). Community motivation must be worked out within the context of local cultures and social structures.[6]

Because communicable diseases interact with other conditions, such as childhood malnutrition, programmes would have to be organized in close collaboration with maternal and child health services. This 'positioning' of immunization as between, or as linking, the 'vertical' and the 'horizontal' was politically vital. Immunization did mean that certain diseases were being singled out, and in that sense could be viewed as embodying the vertical programme favoured by the USA. On the other hand there was an insistence that vaccination should be integrated with primary healthcare, and should indeed be viewed as a means of strengthening it. In other words, it was also an element in the horizontal approach preferred by the Soviet bloc.

In May 1974, as the smallpox campaign was entering its final stages, the World Health Assembly adopted a resolution formally establishing what became known as the Expanded Programme of Immunization, or EPI. Resolution 27.57 recommended member states to 'develop or maintain immunization and surveillance programmes against some or all of the following diseases: diphtheria, pertussis, tetanus, measles, poliomyelitis, tuberculosis, smallpox and others, where applicable, according to the epidemiological situation in their respective countries'. The resolution also requested the director general

> to intensify at all levels of the Organization its activities pertaining to the development of immunization programmes, especially for the developing countries; to assist Member States (i) in developing suitable programmes by providing technical advice on the use of vaccines and (ii) in assuring the availability of good-quality vaccines at reasonable cost; to study the possibilities of providing from international sources and agencies an increased supply of vaccines, equipment and transport and developing local competence to produce vaccines at the national level.[7]

There was certainly a long way to go. Eighty million children were born each year in the African, Latin American and Southeast Asian regions taken together, and of these only some four million were being effectively immunized. The organization's immediate target was to help countries expand the coverage of their immunization programmes, whether geographically or in terms of the number of antigens given.

The view at the WHO was that national governments themselves should take the initiative. No one was going to force them to introduce a particular antigen or to make vaccination a priority. There was no 'one-size-fits-all' perspective. Action would be triggered when an individual country asked the WHO for help in determining whether, and if so how, it could adapt the arrangements put in place in the smallpox eradication programme in order to boost vaccination against the other childhood diseases. The next step would then be for a government that wanted to participate to develop an operational plan. This would be based on a planning exercise in which WHO staff based in the country would participate. The planning should start from demographics and disease epidemiology in the country, and then move on to assess resources available, forms of organization and sociocultural aspects of acceptability. Which vaccines were needed and what were the long-term requirements? Countries would have to establish systems of surveillance and evaluation, to define objectives and requirements, to train personnel and to educate the public regarding the benefits of immunization.

A series of regional seminars was organized. Taking place in Kumasi (Ghana), Damascus (Syria), Manila (Philippines) and Delhi (India), these seminars were intended to encourage countries to participate in the EPI, to explain the planning process and to discuss the technical and organizational problems and choices that they would have to face. For example, how should the vaccines best be delivered? Would it be best to rely on existing clinics providing child health services, carry out vaccination in rural areas with special mobile teams, or use a combination of both? Speakers at these seminars stressed that immunization was to form part of basic health services. Community nurses, especially those in maternal/child care, would have a vital role to play. The expectation, shared in many ministries of health, was that as the smallpox campaign came to an end it should be possible to shift resources to the new programme. To help launch the EPI the WHO turned to UNICEF for support, and in 1975 the two organizations agreed on what was to be a fundamental principle of the new programme. It would be developed gradually and the initiative had to lie with individual countries. This was vital, because vaccination programmes would have to be continued indefinitely, and for this, national commitment was regarded as a *sine qua non*.

By late 1975 a growing number of countries had indicated that they wished to collaborate with the WHO in expanding their immunization programme. In the African region collaboration with Ghana, Kenya, Tanzania and Zambia was already under way. In Ghana and Kenya detailed epidemiological and technical studies were being carried out, with financial support from Sweden and the Netherlands respectively. Studies focused on the specific problems likely to be faced in the particular country, and because health service organization and provision differed widely from country to country, so did the problems likely to be faced. For example, in Ghana the study examined the relative effectiveness of fixed centres and mobile teams for vaccinating small children. Was vaccination of expectant mothers against neonatal tetanus feasible in Ghana? Elsewhere different issues arose, as for example in Mozambique. The country's long war of independence from Portugal had only ended in 1974. The new Mozambique Liberation Front (FRELIMO) government saw a successful vaccination programme as providing a foundation on which general health services could be built. Though the country was in economic disarray, it soon had a three-year project, financed by the United Nations Development Programme (UNDP), which would use mobile teams to vaccinate the whole population against smallpox, measles and tuberculosis. But the project was derailed because in 1977 a civil war broke out, in which anti-government forces were supported by the apartheid regime in South Africa, by the Rhodesians and by the CIA.

How was the Expanded Programme of Immunization to be justified at a time of growing political tension? Beyond the now all too familiar posturing inherent in Cold War discussions, there were the sensitivities of the newly independent states of the 'Global South'. At the 1976 World Health Assembly the delegate from Niger (a former French colony which had become independent in 1958) had this to say: 'One sometimes got the impression that in discussing immunization programmes, people regarded the underdeveloped countries as a reservoir of disease, and gave their assistance primarily to prevent that disease from spreading.' He gave various examples of developing countries not receiving the vaccines they expected, or not on time, or vaccines that, by the time they arrived, were no longer effective. There was a great need of local centres for checking the quality of vaccines: 'Even when they could afford the price, they did not get the product or the advice they required.'[8] And the system was corrupt. There were examples of vaccines being offloaded from a plane to make space for a shipment of munitions.

Many practical issues were still to be resolved if the EPI was to be implemented effectively. One concerned the stability of the vaccines. The smallpox campaign had been successful thanks to the existence of freeze-dried vaccine, which could withstand high temperatures. For most other vaccines, no such freeze-dried version existed. Most of them, including the measles vaccine, were very sensitive to both heat and light. This meant that special means of refrigerated storing and transportation of vaccine would have to be established if the vaccine were still to be potent when delivered to a remote rural area. Setting up a reliable 'cold chain' was going to add significantly to the technical difficulties, and the costs, of developing a comprehensive vaccine programme in any tropical country.

If coverage was to be as high as possible, how should immunization programmes best be organized? Should children receive their vaccine together with other services and support offered by local health centres? Or was a mass campaign likely to be more effective: dispatching mobile teams of vaccinators whose sole job it would be to vaccinate children? Given that resources were limited, the strategy that made most sense could well depend on what was already in place, and this would differ from country to country. In Africa, different colonial traditions in ex-British and ex-French colonies had left newly independent states with quite different healthcare institutions and practices. It was hardly surprising, then, that studies on the cost-effectiveness of different strategies carried out in different countries came to different conclusions. It often seemed that after the successes of the early phases of a mass campaign things began to taper off. Experiences differed from country to country, as one British expert pointed out at the time:

> an evaluation of a measles–smallpox campaign in the Ivory Coast, where mobile vaccination teams visited each village every 12–18 months, showed 54 per cent coverage of children 6–24 months. Poor publicity was considered the main problem here. A measles campaign in Senegal achieved about 60 per cent coverage, and a mobile mass campaign in Yaounde was highly effective for smallpox, but achieved inadequate coverage to control measles.[9]

There was no single best way of organizing and extending an immunization programme. But while improving the effectiveness of programme implementation was a crucial objective, the WHO and its representatives had to tread very carefully in formulating recommendations, or even discussing the EPI. The major commitment to extending and expanding vaccination programmes that the WHO was now making could seem to imply alignment with the vertical approach favoured by the United States. If that was too apparently and too explicitly the case, not only would the Soviet Union be angered, it also conflicted with the direction in which Mahler was trying to move the organization. The result was that WHO staff constantly emphasized that countries should make every effort to integrate immunization programmes with basic health services. They were best seen as providing a foundation on which a system of primary healthcare could be built, as for example the Mozambique government had intended. Senior officials of the organization made the point at every opportunity. Introducing the EPI at a meeting in the African region, the regional director for Africa reminded delegates of the need to integrate vaccination programmes with their country's socio-economic development: 'This activity should be carried out within the national health services structure. The expanded programme on immunization is to be included in the concept of primary healthcare, basic health measures, and integrated rural development.' To achieve its full potential, community leaders would have to be convinced of the vaccination programme's benefits and be actively involved: political and religious leaders, teachers, community leaders and those in charge of development, as well as any person who had a certain influence, should be involved:

> This . . . will require systematic educational action by all personnel carrying out the immunization programme. Before beginning a programme, the target group who will receive the necessary education must be specifically defined and fundamental information gathered about the knowledge of this group, its attitude, beliefs and prejudices towards immunization and the diseases which can be prevented by it. Methods and means of information will then have to be chosen in such a way as to ensure a basic knowledge of all aspects of immunization. The benefits of immunization must not be exaggerated.[10]

In 1977 an ambitious and much more specific goal was established for the EPI. By 1990 every child in the world should receive the standard EPI vaccines (against diphtheria, pertussis, tetanus, poliomyelitis, measles and tuberculosis). Enormous progress was

being made as more and more countries established immunization programmes or increased the scope of existing programmes.
For example, Colombia, where in 1975 only 9 per cent of children
under one year had been immunized with DPT, succeeded in raising
coverage to 75 per cent by 1989. This was achieved thanks to active
political support, and the mobilization of hundreds of teachers,
priests, policemen and Red Cross volunteers in 'national immunization days': a model that, with the enthusiastic support of UNICEF,
was widely adopted.

The rhetoric was sustained into the 1980s. Thus in 1984, EPI's
Geneva-based director, R. H. Henderson, explained that while
immunization services are only part of the answer to reducing
childhood mortality, nevertheless they

> can be a good entry point for the development of other health
> services because they are simple to administer and because
> their effectiveness does not require a complex change in
> attitudes or life-styles on the part of the mother or the child.[11]

He continued by pointing out that while it was perfectly possible to
provide immunization services alone, 'they are best delivered along
with other services needed by children during their first year of life
and by pregnant women – the persons who constitute the priority
groups for primary healthcare services in the developing world.'

Slowly but surely, however, and despite the rhetoric, immunization was in practice being decoupled from primary healthcare
both administratively and organizationally. Meeting coverage targets was becoming more and more important. Simple numbers,
which in international fora could easily be used to show progress,
were becoming more important than the more complex, less easily
quantified ideals that had inspired the Alma Ata declaration. For
officials in international health who still held on to those ideals, a
high level of immunization coverage was not an appropriate measure of progress in healthcare. The criteria against which progress
had to be judged were the overall adequacy of the healthcare system,
popular satisfaction with that system and community influence over
it. Judged in this way, a successful immunization programme could
actually be counterproductive if it drew people and resources away
from basic healthcare:

The accounts which are now becoming available from Africa and Asia of the destructive effects at the district and peripheral levels of the health system by processes such as preferential field allowances to workers participating in vertical EPI programmes are so dramatic that they cannot be ignored.[12]

There was evidence that this is precisely what was happening in some places. Ecuador had been one of the first Latin American countries to introduce the EPI.[13] A conservative president, elected in 1984, was committed to implementing the 'structural-adjustment' policies being forced on poor countries by the World Bank. Looking for a means of mitigating the unpopularity that would accompany these measures, the country's president was receptive to a suggestion from the executive director of UNICEF that he start a mass vaccination effort. With $4 million from the United States Agency for International Development (USAID), the programme would reduce maternal and infant mortality, and would increase rates of immunization against polio, diphtheria and whooping cough. In order to ensure the effectiveness of the initiative, a special administrative structure was established. Not only was its staff better paid than regular Ministry of Health officials, but it gradually escaped control by the ministry: a gradual 'verticalization', in other words. Particular emphasis was placed on the organization of National Immunization Days (NIDS). As the name suggests, these were (and are) a mechanism much favoured by the EPI, in the course of which vaccination teams blanket the country. Seven of these NIDS were organized in Ecuador, supported by massive media promotion. When USAID support ended, in 1989, both administrative organization and routine vaccination programmes had difficulty in taking over responsibility. The cost per vaccination dose in the special campaign proved to have been nearly three times the cost of providing vaccines through routine services. What is more, immediately after the intensive programme ended, numbers of measles cases rose to levels even higher than they had been before the programme started!

Despite the progress, it was becoming clear that the goal of vaccinating every child in the world by 1990 was not going to be achieved without considerable additional resources. Recognizing this, some of the major international organizations active in promoting international health and vaccination met together in 1984. At the meeting, the World Bank, the UNDP and the Rockefeller Foundation joined the WHO and UNICEF in establishing a 'Task Force for Child Survival' (now known as the Task Force for Global Health). William Foege, recently retired as director of the U.S. CDC, was brought in to run it. The task force was to serve as a catalyst, mobilizing support for immunization (and other healthcare initiatives) among international donors. It would also organize a series of meetings to bring the heads of development agencies together with the health ministers of developing countries. One of these meetings, held at Talloires, France, in 1988 was to prove particularly significant, as we will see in the following chapter.

Taking Stock: The Cold War Years

The decades following the end of the Second World War have been called a 'golden age' of scientific discovery, and this was as true of vaccine science as of any other. Enders's research at Harvard led to the development of new vaccines, most significantly against polio and measles, each with the potential to save countless lives and a great deal of suffering. Of course, lives would be saved only if children at risk actually received the vaccine. For this, public health professionals and national policymakers had to be convinced of the value of vaccination, they had to find the necessary human and financial resources, and they had to design appropriate programmes.

By the 1950s, the political map of the world had changed, as a result of decolonization movements across Africa and Asia, and of the emerging Cold War. Cold War rivalries soon began to influence the field of public health, including the politics surrounding vaccination. Neither East nor West wasted any opportunity in trying to convince the non-aligned world of its own technical and moral superiority. The newly established World Health Organization, and its 'parliament', the World Health Assembly, provided an important forum for doing just that. Irrespective of ideological games being played out in public, once the WHO had committed itself to eradicating smallpox, the technical representatives of each side had little difficulty in working together. But the motives of East and West for supporting the campaign in the first place were different. For the Soviet Union and its allies the hope was that a successful campaign would enable costly vaccination to end and resources to be saved. With the malaria campaign failing, the United States needed a new humanitarian mission to help mitigate the damage done to its reputation by the Vietnam War.

Vaccination had become an established tool of preventive health by this time, and there was little of the hesitation that, in some countries, had marked earlier responses to BCG. Because it was a widely feared and devastating disease, few industrialized countries waited very long before deciding to begin polio vaccination, though the start was often triggered in response to a national epidemic. On the other hand, the efficiency with which campaigns could be mounted depended on the organization of public health systems. The greater the degree of centralization and state organization, the easier it was to mount an effective national campaign. There were national differences, even between European countries, but they now reflected a mix of ideological and organizational factors and tradition. There were new measles vaccines in addition to those against polio. Their introduction shows something slightly different, because measles was of far less concern than polio in the industrialized world. Here a difference is to be seen between the United States' response to the measles vaccines and the responses of most European countries. It was partly a matter of timing. It was becoming clear that, in the United States, infectious disease was increasingly concentrated among the poor. For the Kennedy and Johnson administrations, with their new social welfare programmes, this was both embarrassing and unacceptable. Measles vaccination would have to help reduce social disparities. This was less apparently the case in Western Europe, where many countries hesitated before starting measles vaccination. Knowing that few parents thought measles very serious, governments felt it important to assess likely popular demand before embarking on a vaccination campaign. Introducing a vaccine in the face of popular reluctance, policymakers felt, could endanger confidence in the national vaccination programme as a whole. This, above all, had to be avoided.

It was in the developing world where measles vaccine was most needed, as were the vaccines against diphtheria, tuberculosis and whooping cough. These diseases were still killing thousands of children every year in Africa and Asia. At the start of the 1970s, few children in the developing world were vaccinated, other than against smallpox. Building on the smallpox campaign, the new Expanded

Programme of Immunization (EPI) would provide help and advice for countries wishing to establish or extend vaccination against infectious diseases. The EPI was based on the idea that countries would decide their own priorities, and the WHO would advise and assist – not lead or cajole – them. Countries were to develop and extend vaccination against the diseases that most concerned them, and within the general context of their plans for socio-economic development. To the extent feasible, they would be expected to integrate vaccination with the basic healthcare systems that would form part of their development plans. There was little trace, as yet, of a 'one-size-fits-all' approach.

Officials involved with the EPI had to watch their words, because of the extent to which ideological rivalries had permeated public health debates. A clear divide had opened up between those who argued that the way forward involved strengthening primary health-care, and tackling the root causes of disease, and those who favoured using proven weapons (including vaccines) to tackle specific diseases. Though immunization was necessarily against a specific disease, WHO officials consistently emphasized the importance of integrating vacci-nation programmes with other health services. There were, however, tendencies – growing in strength – for vaccination programmes to cut loose, to operate in an increasingly 'vertical' manner, organizationally and administratively. There were critics who noted this with alarm, who argued that a high rate of vaccination coverage was no indicator of the quality of a health system, but they were unheeded.

In May 1980 the WHA adopted a resolution declaring that small-pox had been eradicated from the globe. Widely hailed as public health's greatest triumph, different people drew different lessons from the eradication of smallpox. For one thing, having shown what could be achieved by global leadership and coordination, the campaign had already led to the establishment of the EPI. Other lessons were also drawn. Some saw it as establishing global eradica-tion as a feasible and desirable public health goal. This was a lesson against which the WHO's director general at the time warned the public health community. Historian Anne-Emanuelle Birn reminds us that in 1980 Mahler stressed that 'important lessons can be learned from smallpox eradication – but the idea that we should single out other diseases for worldwide eradication is not among them. That idea is tempting but illusory.'[14]

Yet as we will see in the next chapter, this is precisely the lesson that a few powerful individuals were determined to draw. Some of the most central assumptions that had underpinned policies for deploying vaccines, nationally and internationally, would soon be forgotten or discarded.

SEVEN

POLICIES: VACCINATION IN A GLOBALIZING WORLD

Changing Rationalities

E arlier we saw how the shift in the ideological basis of public policy that took place in the 1980s influenced vaccine development. What now of its effects on the way vaccines were used, on the place of vaccination in healthcare, and on access?

In the 1980s, the u.s. government, and the international organizations it largely dominated, including the World Bank and the International Monetary Fund, began to make their support for poor countries conditional on adherence to principles of deregulation, liberalization and privatization. The role of the state had to be reduced as far as possible. Under the influence of the u.s. Treasury, the World Bank began to make 'structural-adjustment loans', with which desperately indebted countries could pay their debts and keep services running. In the health field, these loans were becoming vital to the ability of many poor countries to provide even basic health services. Stringent conditions were attached, however. Health services would have to be privatized, decentralized and deregulated. Users would be required to pay fees. A few governments, such as Chile's Pinochet dictatorship, were innately sympathetic to these economic ideas and soon restructured their health services accordingly. Others reacted more reluctantly, though few were able wholly to avoid cutbacks in publicly provided health services. In much of the world it became more and more difficult for poor families to obtain formal healthcare. As these measures took hold things got worse. Malaria, for example, claimed well over a million lives each year in the 1980s: largely the lives of African children. As the restructuring required by international donors took hold, the malaria death rate in southern Africa actually rose. Not that it was only malaria that claimed the lives of hundreds of thousands of children in poor countries. Pneumonia was responsible for 10 per cent of all children's deaths in the developing world. Another major risk came from lack of access to pure drinking water. In places with poor sanitation and polluted water supplies, communities are exposed to pathogens causing diarrhoeal disease. Once again, children are most likely to suffer. Rotavirus caused serious diarrhoeal disease among something like two million children a year, and more than 450,000 under-fives died each year as a result. *Shigella* caused millions of cases of severe dysentery annually, with at least 100,000 of these resulting in death, again mostly among children in the developing world.

The idea that the 'market knows best', which became so influential in the era of Reagan and Thatcher, brought with it a major redistribution of authority. By the end of the millennium, the multinational pharmaceutical industry enjoyed far greater influence than it had before, while governments were far more constrained in their actions. New philanthropic organizations, notably the Bill and Melinda Gates Foundation, brought considerable new resources into public health – as well as a particular set of values. How did these developments influence recourse to vaccines as a tool of public health? That is the question for this chapter. In fact, however, the roots of the changes taking place are to be found earlier, in the 1970s. It was in the latter part of that decade that the rapidly rising costs of healthcare began to worry politicians, with unbridled recourse to expensive new technologies seemingly a major contributory factor. This was the moment when economists stepped in, and persuaded policymakers that they, and they alone, had the tools with which difficult but unavoidable choices could be made rationally.

Unlike polio, rubella and mumps are not killer diseases. Unlike measles, they are not, and were not even in the 1970s, major threats to the health of children in poor countries. Many African and Asian countries do not include mumps and rubella antigens in their vaccination schedules even now. But children born in North America, Australia or Europe are expected to be vaccinated against both when they are twelve to fifteen months old, with a booster shot following a few years later. The start of rubella and mumps vaccination shows how new considerations were becoming important in formulating vaccination policy.

Developments in public health have always reflected the outcome of political negotiations, whether focused on priorities,
influence, economic interests or the assertion of national independence. Like a work of art or a scientific paper, the final product – a
policy – should conceal the difficult work of its construction. Public
health policies are explained and justified differently to different
publics and in different arenas. It depends on what is at stake. For
example, as we saw in the previous chapter, during the Cold War
success in disease control was a field in which East and West each
tried to show its technological and ideological superiority. But to
parents, vaccines and vaccination programmes are presented as
tools for the protection of their child, for the avoidance of needless
risks to its health. And of course they are that, though not that alone.
Vaccination policy involves more than simply the decision to provide, or not to provide, a particular vaccine. For example, decisions
will have to be made as to who should receive the vaccine, how many
doses they will need and when, and who should be first in line if the
vaccine is in short supply. Moreover, if we look behind the scenes, at
the way decisions are arrived at, we see a slightly different logic at
play. On what basis are these decisions made? The start of mumps
and rubella vaccinations shows how by the 1970s goals in addition to
the protection of individual children were exerting increasing influence. Of course, in public pronouncements protection of the child
always has to be emphasized, since parents will not take their child
to be immunized in order to save healthcare money or to eradicate
a disease. (Whether they'll do so in the interests of the community
as a whole is a moot point, and one to which the answer probably
differs from place to place.) In this chapter we will see a gap emerging between the logic of policymaking on the one hand, and public
perceptions of vaccination policy on the other. This gap is growing,
with consequences that we will discuss in the final chapter.

When rubella vaccination was being considered, in the 1970s, it
was recognized that the nature of the disease meant that it posed a
distinctive challenge. Rubella (German measles) is not so serious for
the person who catches it, but if that person happens to be pregnant
the results can be very serious. It was a foetus as yet unconceived
that needed protection, not the woman bearing it. How was the
vaccine to be used? Vaccinating young women of childbearing age
directly, with a (potentially teratogenic) live-virus vaccine, was felt

to be too dangerous. But if the vaccine were to be given to children (who are easier to reach) it was essential that the immunity it provided would last through a possible pregnancy years later.

When rubella vaccination started, most European countries offered the vaccine to girls only, since it was they who ran the risk of rubella-related foetal malformations. The vaccine would have to be administered well before there was any possibility of their being pregnant. This was the strategy followed in the Netherlands, so that, starting in 1974, eleven-year-old girls were vaccinated against rubella. Reported cases fell from roughly two to three thousand per year in the early 1970s to roughly seven to eight hundred in the years thereafter. However, a crucial uncertainty remained. Would protection conferred on young girls persist until the time of an eventual pregnancy? Not much was known about the duration of protection that the vaccine provided.

Reasoning differently, public health authorities in the United States had decided to vaccinate all young children. The best strategy would be to establish herd immunity among children, for it was among children that these viruses mainly circulated. If the virus had been more or less eliminated, pregnant women would be protected indirectly. Despite encouraging trends, it was hardly plain sailing. This was partly because the u.s. couldn't achieve the high vaccination rates that many European countries managed. Community-level studies showed that even vaccination rates of 80 or 90 per cent did not block introduction and transmission of the rubella virus. Experience with other vaccines suggested that, in the usa, overall rates of much above 60–70 per cent would be difficult to achieve.

The United Kingdom adopted the same strategy as the Netherlands. Starting in 1970, rubella vaccine was offered to schoolgirls aged eleven to thirteen. Like the Dutch they had considered the American strategy but had rejected it, mainly because measles vaccination coverage at the time was only around 50 per cent and there were fears that a universal strategy would be unsuccessful. Though there were some schoolgirls who refused the vaccine, coverage quickly reached 78 per cent (rising to 86 per cent by 1988). Reports of congenital rubella syndrome (crs), terminations of pregnancy related to rubella infection and laboratory studies of pregnant women all showed trends in the right direction. By the late 1980s there were estimated to be 22 births of rubella syndrome-affected children in a year, while 73 pregnancies were terminated because of it.

The risk to a vaccinated woman who might later become pregnant depended on the length of time for which the vaccine conferred protection, as well as on the extent to which live virus continued to circulate. This second factor itself depended on the degree of coverage achieved. In other words, the longer the duration of protection and the more people vaccinated, the lower the risk to any individual. In the United Kingdom, simulation modelling was becoming an important new input into the study of infectious diseases. Introducing values for how infectious a given pathogen was believed to be (the R_0 we met earlier) and how protective a vaccine, computer models were being used to predict the future spread of diseases. A simulation study of rubella suggested that the best strategy would depend on the efficacy of the vaccine, on uptake rates and on the rate of decay in immunity over time, but also on the relative importance to be attached to short-term benefits as against the risk of subsequent resurgence. In the light of this, it could not be taken for granted that the optimal strategy in a country with high coverage would be the best strategy for one with low coverage. Crucially, however, the very purpose of rubella vaccination in Europe was about to change. Instead of offering direct protection to the individual woman, the objective of rubella vaccination was now to be halting circulation of the virus. This was the objective on which policy in the United States had been based from the start. The Americans had been right in concluding that by vaccinating girls only it would not be possible to eliminate the virus to stop its circulation.

As in the UK, the Netherlands' selective strategy had considerably reduced the incidence of rubella-related foetal malformations and pregnancy terminations. However, health-policy advisers noted the British conclusion that it couldn't actually prevent them totally. Intrigued by the British simulation study, the Dutch Health Council wished to repeat it using data from the Netherlands. Feeding available data into a simulation model suggested that the combined strategy would be best for the Netherlands. More specifically, it appeared that if both boys and girls were vaccinated at the age of fourteen months and girls again at the age of eleven years, the rubella virus could be eliminated with a coverage rate of 85 per cent. If both boys *and* girls were vaccinated for a second time at the age of nine this would be the case with a coverage rate of 75 per cent. Somehow, elimination of the virus had now become the objective, and in 1983 the Dutch minister of health was advised to replace the current rubella strategy by one in which both boys and girls would be vaccinated at the age of twelve months and again at nine years. The expectation was that this would lead to the virtual elimination of rubella within five to ten years. (Computer simulation models also suggested that rubella could well become *more* prevalent within the small communities opposed to vaccination on religious grounds. Government advisers felt this was no reason to question a strategy deemed to be in the interest of the majority.)

By the mid-1980s the majority of European countries had followed the United States in switching to universal rubella vaccination, with only a handful of countries (including the UK and Ireland) still hesitating. In the UK the need for a change of strategy was being debated with an eye on what other countries were doing. For example, in 1986 three Scottish public health specialists wrote in the *British Medical Journal*:

> There is an excellent case for combining measles, mumps and rubella immunisation at 15–18 months of age as is currently done in the United States and several other countries. By adopting such a policy in 1982 Sweden has shown that the complete eradication of measles, mumps and rubella is entirely practicable.[1]

In most European countries babies were vaccinated against rubella at the age of twelve to eighteen months. This was followed (depending on the country) either by a second universal vaccination at six to twelve years, or else a second vaccination of girls only between the ages of ten and fifteen. Simulation modelling had shown that elimination of congenital rubella syndrome using the 'selective' approach would only be possible if all susceptible women were vaccinated using a 100 per cent effective vaccine. Few vaccines are 100 per cent effective. Vaccination schedules in Europe were becoming more and more standardized. An important argument now put forward by advisers on vaccination policy was that increasing mobility in Europe made standardization essential, and that this was particularly so as far as susceptible young women were concerned.

Countries changed their rubella vaccination strategies either because they became convinced that the goal should be to eliminate the virus, rather than to protect potential mothers directly, or because they felt a need to do as neighbouring countries were doing. But what about mumps? Mumps threatened neither children's lives nor the well-being of future generations. It was widely regarded as a mild children's disease, if anything slightly comical on account of the swollen glands it caused. So why did so many countries, including the Netherlands and the UK, start vaccinating children against mumps?

A *Lancet* editorial published a few months after Merck's mumps vaccine was licensed in the USA noted that there had been no suggestion of introducing mumps vaccination in the UK. Since there was no obligation on doctors to report cases of mumps, there was little information on how common it was. A survey of general practitioners found that orchitis (an infection of the testes) complicated about 9 per cent of cases of mumps in boys aged fourteen or over. Though painful this could be relieved by cortico-steroids. Widespread popular belief notwithstanding, sterility was very rare indeed. Aseptic meningitis developed in 2.4 per cent of cases, and although this too was usually followed by complete recovery, it did mean that the patient was admitted to hospital. Approximately 1,300 patients per annum were admitted to hospital with mumps, mainly on account of aseptic meningitis. In the Netherlands, where from 1976 onwards doctors were required to report cases of mumps, there were roughly one thousand cases per year. Almost all of these were among children of less than nine years of age, and complications, which were rare, were almost always treated successfully. In the decade of 1968–78, a total of 48 deaths were attributed to mumps in the Netherlands, more than half of them in middle-aged and elderly patients. In England and Wales, 93 deaths were recorded as due to mumps between 1962 and 1981, mostly among people aged over 45. Inspection of death certificates suggested that many of these deaths were not in fact due to mumps.[2]

While the Merck vaccine appeared to lack side effects and seemed to work for at least two years, was it needed? Was it necessary, or indeed desirable, to try to prevent so mild a disease? The medical profession was in two minds. In a 1969 editorial *The*

Lancet noted, 'The faultless performance of the vaccine in these early trials will raise hopes that mumps can be easily and safely eradicated from a community.' On the other hand, the editorial continued, '[Professor George] Dick has rightly warned, however, that more and more virus vaccines should not be foisted upon us just because it is possible to make them.'[3] A 1980 editorial in the *British Medical Journal* questioned the public's likely response. 'Unless the ill-founded but commonly held dread of sterility from mumps orchitis overcomes the British distrust of new vaccines,' the *Journal* wrote, 'the acceptance rate would almost certainly be low.'[4] Moreover, there was the risk that if protection wore off after a few years, there might be more mumps among adults, for whom it was more serious. The dominant view, in early 1980s Britain, was totally different from that expressed by Langmuir in the USA, to the effect that 'if it could be done then it should be done'. Similarly, in the Netherlands mumps was seen as a minor disease of childhood. It received little attention in the Dutch medical press. When Merck's European subsidiary, MSD, applied for permission to import Mumpsvax to the Netherlands, in 1971, the government saw no reason to deny permission. But nor was there any reason to consider mass vaccination against mumps.

Public and professional perceptions of the severity of mumps had initially been no different in the United States, which did not bode well for the vaccine's commercial prospects. If it were to be a success, people would have to learn to see mumps differently. What happened thereafter, as historian Elena Conis has nicely shown, is that mumps, like measles earlier, though with greater difficulty, was 'rebranded' for the American public.[5] Conis shows how reports inspired by the new vaccine increasingly emphasized risks of brain damage and mental retardation, despite the fact that these risks had been neither quantified nor proven. In other fora mumps was dubbed a 'nuisance', an 'inconvenience' that American parents no longer had to tolerate. Mumps, as Conis puts it, was 'rhetorically transformed' into a serious disease of children, gradually moving from 'nuisance to be avoided' to 'deadly crippler'.[6]

It is easy to see the importance of 'rebranding' in a health system oriented to its fee-paying customers, and where the direct advertising of drugs and vaccines to the public is permitted and common. In Europe the direct advertising of drugs and vaccines is not permitted, so no such marketing campaign would be possible. If the public perception of a disease was going to have to be changed then it would have to be done differently. So how did government advisers become committed to the idea of vaccinating against a disease that was generally felt to be trivial? What arguments, or what evidence, convinced them?

When the Dutch Health Council, responding to a request from the minister of health, began to discuss mumps vaccination, members disagreed as to what evidence was most relevant. Mumps in children was relatively innocuous, and mumps-related mortality was minimal. Moreover, little was known about the duration of protection that the vaccination would provide. There was a risk of circulation being shifted to older age groups. But some members pointed to the fact that the vaccine was already being used in the USA, Germany and Sweden. A representative of the government Health Inspectorate noted the likelihood that the European Parliament would recommend harmonization of vaccination schedules in Europe. Mumps vaccination was a principal difference between schedules in different European countries. Economic arguments were introduced. They suggested that the cost of providing the vaccine would be less than the costs associated with the hospital admission of mumps patients. Other things being equal, money could be saved. Looking at the numbers of people admitted to hospital with mumps, and the lengths of stay, the Health Inspectorate had estimated that in 1979 these hospital costs had been twice what had been spent on measles vaccine. The duration of protection provided and the consequent risk of enhanced virus circulation among older age groups remained a source of uncertainty. Available data were inadequate for mathematical modelling to be of much value.

The sense that this was an unimportant disease was gradually overridden by three considerations. One was practice elsewhere. Dutch advisers were impressed by data from the USA showing an enormous fall in the number of reported cases of mumps. Second, and different, was a growing sense that the Dutch vaccination schedule would *have* to be harmonized with those of other European countries as a result of EU policy initiatives. And third was money. Although data for much more than a back-of-the-envelope calculation were not available, potential savings to the healthcare budget figured largely in the committee's discussions. These were the considerations that were now crucial: saving money, and harmonization. But who should be vaccinated? It was boys who were the more susceptible and adult men who faced particular (though very slight) risks. Nevertheless, in 1983 the Dutch minister of health was advised that *all* children should be vaccinated against mumps at the age of fourteen months (with a second shot later). The reason had to do with the fact that everyone else was switching to the combined MMR vaccine that Merck had introduced. Vaccinating boys only was incompatible with use of the combined vaccine, which would have to be given to all children. So, in order to muster support among parents, arguments for vaccinating girls would have to be found. Policy advisers came up with the following arguments. First, that a 'significant' number of girls were also admitted to hospital with mumps (in fact an average of 115 per annum). A second argument was that vaccinating only boys (in other words, half the children) would insufficiently reduce virus circulation, so that passive protection of the non-immunized would be limited.

In 1986 the Dutch minister of health decided to introduce MMR to the national vaccination programme. He justified his decision by reference to studies conducted elsewhere, undeterred by the lack of cost-effectiveness studies carried out in the Netherlands itself. This statement points to more than the overriding importance that economic evidence had now acquired. It hints also at a shift in the relative weight coming to be attached to national as against international evidence. Twenty years later these would be dominant elements in decision-making (though not in public discussion). If a vaccine had been shown to be effective in one place then it could be assumed to be effective in another even when no studies had been conducted there. The only reason for hesitation would be when circulating virus strains were clearly very different. In 1988 mumps vaccination began in the UK too.

The Eradication Drive

In the course of the 1980s, not only were economic arguments becoming increasingly important, but so was the view that vaccination programmes should aim not merely at controlling disease but at 'eliminating' viruses. While this idea caught on slowly in Europe, in the United States it had a longer history and far more traction.[7]

In 1980 a meeting took place at the National Institutes of Health in Bethesda, Maryland. Drawing its inspiration from the smallpox eradication campaign, and consciously ignoring Mahler's warning that this was not the lesson to be drawn, the meeting's organizers were determined to identify future eradication targets, as historian William Muraskin has shown.[8] Two of the principal architects of smallpox eradication, Frank Fenner and D. A. Henderson, argued that there simply were no feasible eradication targets. Well, one would have to be found. Measles and polio were put forward as the most likely candidates. It mattered less what was eradicated: what was essential was that the smallpox campaign be followed up. In 1982 a paper arguing for the desirability and the feasibility of measles eradication appeared in *The Lancet*.[9] Its authors, all from the CDC, were convinced that measles could be not only controlled, but actually eradicated, if vaccine was widely and properly used. The case for doing so was clear, since measles cost 900,000 lives each year. And it could be done, just as smallpox eradication had been, thanks to the more heat-stable vaccines that were becoming available. Should eradication, rather than control, be the goal? Not everyone was convinced. Meanwhile, the preference of the CDC eradicationists was swinging towards polio rather than measles. At a symposium on polio control which took place in Washington, DC, in 1983, almost no participants spoke in favour of a polio eradication campaign. Polio was not a major public health concern in the developing world, and 'control' was a more appropriate goal. Again, this did not seem to matter.

In 1985 the Pan American Health Organization (PAHO), which represents the WHO in the Americas, committed itself to the eradication of polio in the region by 1990. The organization had been convinced to do so by Ciro de Quadros, a charismatic epidemiologist from Brazil who had worked on the smallpox eradication campaign in Africa. His objective, according to Muraskin, was to use polio eradication as a means of strengthening health systems, and specifically EPI programmes, in Latin American countries. (This was despite the fact that the head of the EPI at the WHO headquarters was opposed to a polio eradication campaign.) D. A. Henderson agreed to act as technical adviser to the PAHO programme, believing that though global eradication was not feasible, eradication in the Americas was. Moreover, such a goal, he believed, would attract political support for improved disease surveillance systems. In 1987 de Quadros, W. H. Foege, who headed the new Task Force for Child Survival based at the Carter Center in Atlanta, and four senior CDC staff, published an article in the *Bulletin of the World Health Organization* entitled 'The Case for Global Eradication of Poliomyelitis'.[10] Eradication is defined as the 'interruption of transmission of a disease (and the elimination of the causative agent)', with such a low risk of the causative agent being reintroduced 'that preventive measures (e.g. immunization) are no longer required'. Almost all the article deals with 'how' polio eradication should be achieved. Specifically, it argues that the emphasis should be on 'blitzing' through national vaccination days. In much of the world, routine health services would not be adequate and could not be relied upon. The idea that vaccination should be integrated with routine healthcare, so vital to the earlier presentations of the EPI, has been not so much forgotten as specifically rejected. As for 'why' polio should be eradicated, it is taken as self-evident. There is little more than the claim that it should lead to 'strengthening the development of general immunization and primary care services throughout the world' – for which no evidence is presented. 'Global eradication of poliomyelitis is inevitable,' they say, the only question being when it would happen. Their view was an optimistic one: 'Global eradication could be achieved as early as 1995.'[11]

Within a year of this paper's publication, these men had succeeded in engineering a global commitment to polio eradication. In 1988 Foege's Task Force for Child Survival organized a high-level meeting in Talloires (France) to discuss global health priorities for the 1990s. Foege and UNICEF executive director James Grant made clear their support for global polio eradication. Even outgoing director general Halfdan Mahler seems to have been convinced by experience in the Americas, despite continuing resistance from the head of the EPI. In the Declaration of Talloires resulting from the meeting, polio eradication headed the list of global health goals for the 1990s. Just two months later, and despite Mahler's earlier warning, in 1988 the World Health Assembly passed a resolution committing the organization to 'the Eradication of Polio by the year 2000'.[12]

In 1994 the Americas were declared free of wild polio virus. For some, experience there provided a clear proof of feasibility, and a demonstration of what could be achieved globally. But not everyone was so sure. It was by no means clear that all governments would show the same commitment as those of Latin American countries. Moreover, the eradication campaigns in Latin America proved to have had effects that went beyond elimination of polio. They had consequences for health systems more generally. Some eradication enthusiasts had seen the campaign as likely to bring additional resources and additional efficiency to the organization of health services. This did indeed appear to be the case, but only in the better-off countries with well-established health systems. In poorer countries in the region, in which health services were more fragile, there was evidence that a major eradication effort could drain resources from other much-needed services.

In countries where wild polio virus still circulated, the global campaign aimed at ensuring that every child received at least three doses of oral polio vaccine (OPV). Organizationally, there would be national immunization days in which all under-fives would be given supplementary doses of vaccine, and there would be house-to-house OPV 'mop-up' campaigns, targeting areas in which transmission of wild polio virus persisted. It soon became clear that National Immunization Days (NIDS) and the 'mop-up' activities would demand a vast investment of labour. Anthropologist Svea Closser's detailed study of how the campaign works in Pakistan shows just how vast is the investment.[13] A single nationwide campaign, in which thirty million children have to be vaccinated, employs not just the handful of WHO and UNICEF employees in the country but an additional 200,000 workers. In India it is an order of magnitude larger, involving 2.3 million vaccinators and nearly 170 million under-fives.

Despite the investments and a dramatic reduction in cases of polio reported, 'eradication by the year 2000' proved unattainable. Indeed, by that year polio was still found in 23 countries, in nine of which it remained endemic. In 2005, by which time $4 billion had been spent (twice the initial estimate), there were still nearly two thousand cases reported, from sixteen nations. In Afghanistan, India, Nigeria and Pakistan, polio remained endemic, and it was being exported to other countries by travellers.

Why was it proving so much more difficult to eradicate than smallpox had been? One reason concerned the nature of the disease. In anyone who had contracted smallpox, the symptoms were obvious: there were no subclinical cases. By contrast, for every person with paralytic polio there were one to two hundred with no visible symptoms, but who carried the virus and could infect others. Smallpox eradication was achieved with a single shot. However, the polio vaccine is less effective in poor tropical regions, possibly because other related viruses that had infected a child compete with the vaccine in the gut. The consequence is that it takes as many as ten shots to ensure immunity in an Indian or Pakistani child. Closser's detailed ethnographic study of the campaign in Pakistan provides a sense of the difficulties the campaign faces. Nomadic families, for example, are very difficult to follow up. How can one ensure that their children receive ten shots at the requisite time intervals? It is virtually impossible to record coverage in areas, such as shanty towns, that are scarcely mapped. There were areas inhabited by ethnically different people and felt to be so dangerous that female vaccinators were scared to enter. But because they were sure that they would lose their jobs and meagre wages if they admitted to having skipped such areas, they cheated. There were supply problems. Sometimes no vaccine arrived on the day a particular neighbourhood was scheduled for mop-up operations.

As the campaign dragged on for year after year, with one deadline after another passing, fatigue and disillusionment set in. Closser found that many of the community-level vaccinators were disgruntled over pay, and their superiors were increasingly disillusioned. Too many resources were being diverted from other things, including routine immunization, that were more important. After all, polio was not a major threat to the health of Pakistani children. Moreover there was a growing feeling that if it hadn't been eradicated after ten years of sustained effort, it probably never would be. And for the national government, faced with natural disasters, power struggles, the Taliban and much else, polio eradication hardly deserved special attention.

The governments of poor and weak countries cannot risk the anger of the powerful donors driving the polio eradication programme. But a number of international experts have argued that the whole campaign was a mistake from the start. In 2006, three of these, including Isao Arita, who had directed the campaign that eliminated the virus from the WHO's western Pacific region, and Frank Fenner, who had played a leading role in the smallpox campaign, published an article in the journal *Science*. Under the headline 'Is Polio Eradication Realistic?' these eminent public health experts discussed why polio eradication was proving far more difficult than smallpox eradication had been.[14] The smallpox campaign had taken only ten years, while even in 2006 the polio campaign had dragged on for eighteen years. It is impossible to sustain enthusiasm and resources for so long. 'Should the WHO proceed with its current global eradication program, in view of all the difficulties and uncertainties?' Their answer, in 2006, was 'no.' Instead of eradication, the more realistic goal of 'control' should be adopted, and the polio programme should be integrated in the Global Immunization, Vision and Strategy, announced by the WHO in 2005. D. A. Henderson, who had directed the smallpox campaign, was another who argued in public that polio eradication was simply not feasible.

Leaders of the eradication campaign were not, and are still not, deterred, despite costs rising beyond anything anyone ever imagined (or at least, admitted to having imagined). Their response, according to Closser, has been to ignore criticism, to minimize difficulties and endlessly to emphasize the progress being made. Scepticism on the part of donors was the biggest worry, and the critique of leading figures like Arita, Fenner and Henderson was a threat. The optimistic messages coming out of the WHO are not merely part of a strategy designed to ensure that donors don't pull out. People involved at the highest levels in the WHO and in Rotary International, which has played a major role in ensuring the continuation of the programme, genuinely believe in eradication. Their conviction that polio eradication is around the corner seems to be a kind of faith. In matters like that, in matters of faith, critical analysis or suggestions of alternatives simply carry no weight.

As I write, the expectation is that eradication will have been achieved by 2018. Eradication, by the way, has been redefined. Here it is taken to mean 'no new cases', not the definition of eradication ('no further need for immunization') given by the proselytizing eradicationists of the 1980s. No one now doubts that vaccination will have to be continued after 2018, using a new inactivated (Salk-type) vaccine to ensure that there is no spread of vaccine-derived virus. If eradication (even in today's sense) is indeed achieved in 2018, it will have taken thirty years – three times as long as smallpox eradication. Smallpox eradication cost $100 million in international funds (at 1980 prices). Some $10 billion has already been spent on polio eradication, and by 2018 it is estimated that more than $15 billion will have been spent. To bolster its case and ensure continued donor support, the Global Polio Eradication Programme (GPEI) has developed an economic argument, and a model, showing how much money will be saved in the long term.

Svea Closser's study also provides fascinating insight into the programme's political realities. Whose programme is the GPEI? In Pakistan, the pretence is maintained that it is a programme of the Pakistan Ministry of Health, with WHO and UNICEF representatives present only as advisers. Yet it is these advisers who dominate strategy meetings. Though the campaign is based on a resolution passed by the World Health Assembly in 1988, it is no longer exactly a WHO programme either. As its website explains, the GPEI is 'a public–private partnership led by national governments and spearheaded by the World Health Organization (WHO), Rotary International, the U.S. Centers for Disease Control and Prevention (CDC), and the United Nations Children's Fund (UNICEF).' It has its own management and policymaking structure. There is an 'Oversight Board', consisting of the heads of the WHO, UNICEF, the CDC and Rotary (and the head of the Gates Foundation's Global Development Program), chaired, as of September 2015, by the director of the CDC. Much of the work is delegated to an executive Strategy Committee, which meets every two weeks via videoconferencing. Its chair and vice chair are from the WHO and Rotary International respectively, while the heads of polio programmes at the core agencies also participate. There is also a Polio Partners Group, which should meet twice annually at a senior (though lower) level, to 'foster greater engagement among polio-affected countries, donors and other partners with the objective of utilizing their political, communications, programmatic and financial capabilities to ensure GPEI has the necessary political commitment and financial resources to reach the goal of polio eradication.' Country representatives, and representatives of other potential donors or NGOs working in the polio eradication field, might be invited to attend. In a structure like this, both responsibilities and accountability are elusive, and hard to pin down.

Just as the successful smallpox campaign inspired a few determined eradicationists to launch the polio eradication initiative, GPEI in its turn is being used as a launching pad for new eradication initiatives, despite the fact that it has not yet succeeded. When polio eradication is achieved (failure is not contemplated), the campaign will continue with a similar organizational model, but a different target disease. The targets being promoted, notably malaria and measles, have been on the agenda before. The United States launched the world on a malaria eradication drive in the early 1950s, before imminent failure led them to switch to smallpox. CDC epidemiologists have been dreaming of eradicating measles for decades, almost since a measles vaccine became available. In 1996 the CDC hosted a meeting, co-sponsored with the WHO and PAHO, on measles eradication. Participants at that meeting were convinced that global measles eradication was feasible, and that a global eradication campaign, with a target date somewhere between 2005 and 2010 (!), should 'build on the successes of the global Poliomyelitis Eradication Initiative'. They also agreed that for the campaign to be successful measles would have to be 'rebranded' for parents in the industrialized world:

> Measles is often mistakenly perceived as a mild illness. This misperception, which is particularly prevalent in industrialized countries, can inhibit the development of public and political support for the allocation of resources required for an effective elimination effort. . . . The disease burden imposed by measles should be documented, particularly in industrialized countries, so that this information can be used to educate parents, medical practitioners, public health workers, and political leaders about the benefits of measles eradication.[15]

As we saw earlier, Merck had recognized this when first marketing their vaccine in the USA.

Despite occasionally serious local outbreaks, the number of measles deaths across the world has been falling for years, from more than 500,000 deaths in 2000 to fewer than 150,000 in 2010 (overwhelmingly in Africa and Asia). In 2010, the World Health Assembly committed to reducing measles deaths by 95 per cent of the 2000 numbers by 2015. (The actual reduction, between 2000 and 2014, was 79 per cent.) For eradicationists, however, control is not enough, and nor are they willing to await the successful conclusion of the GPEI. A 2012 Global Measles and Rubella Strategic Plan proposed that by the end of 2015 a target date for eradication should have been set, and measles should have been eliminated from five of the six WHO regions by 2020. Scientists agree that, technically speaking, measles eradication is feasible, albeit more difficult than polio eradication. If there is one lesson to be learned from the polio campaign, surely it is that the major problems are social, political and organizational, not scientific. The consequences of an eradication programme for healthcare provision more generally have been shown to vary greatly from place to place. But while global policymakers may have become slightly more cautious than they were thirty years ago, there seems little ability or willingness to take objections seriously.

In contrast to measles, few experts believe in the technical feasibility of malaria eradication, at least with existing tools. Malaria still claims half a million lives each year, most of them in Africa. There is a global malaria-control programme, with an entity called 'Roll Back Malaria' in existence since 1998. Launched by the WHO, UNICEF, the UNDP and the World Bank, its goal is to coordinate control of the disease. Today the programme involves something like five hundred partner organizations, and an expenditure of $2–3 billion per year, which goes on treatments, insecticide-sprayed bed nets and diagnostic tests. Forty years after the previous malaria eradication campaign was aborted, Bill and Melinda Gates have put it back on the global agenda. There is talk of a strategy different from that tried before, and based on gradual elimination, control and surveillance. In 2008 a panel of experts convened by the WHO concluded that stopping transmission would be feasible in low-transmission countries with well-functioning health services (and thus not those countries in which it is most serious). The major problem, the experts recognized, is that vaccination would have to be maintained for years after malaria has ceased to be a major public health concern. Can political commitment be sustained, and will donors continue to provide resources?

New Times, New Priorities, New Processes

Over the past three decades public–private partnerships like GPEI have blossomed. The WHO no longer has the key role, nor the standing, that it once had. In the 1980s the spread of neo-liberal ideologies, and belief in the free play of market forces, meant that authority increasingly reflected financial muscle rather than moral standing. The World Bank, with far greater resources, was increasingly involving itself in reshaping national health systems, while the WHO's continuing commitment to the extension of basic healthcare fitted ill with the 'Washington Consensus'. The pharmaceutical industry, increasingly influential in the new ideological regime, was hardly enamoured of an organization forbidden by its constitution to collaborate with industry. The GPEI is just one of the new institutional structures based on partnerships between public- and private-sector institutions.

The Children's Vaccine Initiative (CVI), established in 1990, pioneered the model in the vaccine field. It was to stimulate the development of new and better vaccines, ultimately of a universal vaccine containing all the antigens the world's children required. But in the course of the following ten years, unbridgeable disagreements emerged between the CVI's European and American donors. Despite shifting its focus from development of new vaccines to supporting vaccine introduction, the CVI was closed down in 1999. Out of its ashes emerged, phoenix-like, a new institution with far greater resources. The Global Alliance for Vaccines and Immunization, now known as the GAVI Alliance, was announced at the 2000 Davos World Economic Forum. Among the principal sponsors of what has since become the dominant force in vaccine policy are the Bill and Melinda Gates Foundation and the International Federation of Pharmaceutical Manufacturers Associations. The GAVI Alliance has become the key actor in articulating and implementing a global vaccine policy, and one which emphasizes the introduction of new vaccines.

Having been evaluated and licensed, how are new vaccines actually introduced into national immunization programmes? There are now many new vaccines, most of which, unlike the old vaccines, are expensive. Adding a vaccine costing tens or even hundreds of euros per shot to a national immunization programme obviously represents a significant public expenditure for any country. Although the final decision generally lies with a minister of health, many countries have some kind of expert committee that advises the minister either in response to a request for advice or at their own initiative. In a number of countries, these have developed decision frameworks, sets of criteria supposedly used in deciding whether a given vaccine should be introduced.

In the United States it is the Advisory Committee on Immunization Practices (ACIP) that has this advisory function, and in the UK it is the Joint Committee on Vaccination and Immunisation (JCVI). The JCVI's tasks include reviewing reports of adverse events related to particular vaccines, and looking ahead: keeping an eye on vaccines likely to come onto the market in the medium term. When a recommendation relating to a new vaccine has to be prepared, a special committee is established to review mortality and morbidity data relating to the disease in question and data on the vaccine. The committee might commission some mathematical modelling designed to capture any herd-immunity effects, and possibly some economic analysis as well. Finally, a subcommittee provides an estimate of the cost-effectiveness of the new vaccine, and makes its recommendation. A vaccine will be recommended, so it is said, if and only if its cost will be less than £2,000–£3,000 per quality-adjusted life year (QALY) gained. Only costs to the health system, and not costs (such as time off work) borne by the family, are taken into account. On the basis of all this the subcommittee reports to the JCVI, and this then sends its recommendation to the minister of health.

It all seems totally rational. Decisions regarding a change to the national immunization programme appear to follow simply and rationally from the objective application of clear criteria, free of bias, lobbying or ideology. With more and more vaccines becoming available, the need not only to choose, but also to justify choices politically, is becoming all the greater. Little wonder that similar decision models have been produced in other industrialized countries. In poor countries it is generally somewhat different, not least because similarly detailed epidemiological data are often not available. Moreover, lacking the financial resources needed to introduce the expensive new vaccines that the WHO recommends, governments look for help. Here is where GAVI comes in. Countries with a per capita annual income of no more than $1,580 (there are 54 of them at present) can apply for GAVI support for new vaccine introduction. They need to prepare a proposal according to its rules, but there is a good chance that the alliance will send an expert to help them prepare it.

When advisers, or the civil servants who prepare policy based on their recommendations, are interviewed – anonymously, of course – the picture that emerges is less objective and rational than written descriptions of the process suggest. The decision to introduce a new vaccine is often a far more political one, in which many considerations other than disease burden, or even cost, play a role. What industrial or strategic interests are involved? What lobbying is going on? How are representatives of international organizations involved (as advocates or advisers) in the policymaking process? Just as happened previously with polio vaccination, a disease outbreak can generate social and political pressure that triggers action. For example, a study by an international group of researchers led by the London School of Hygiene and Tropical Medicine found that diarrhoea outbreaks, which in Guatemala and South Africa gained substantial media attention, led to pressure on ministers of health, as a result of which rotavirus vaccine was introduced.[16] There have not been many studies that give insight into how decisions are actually made in practice, and the few that there are offer a less than reassuring picture. How do doctors and officials who have been involved in deciding on the introduction of a new vaccine explain the process? One thing that becomes clear is that people and institutions that you would think would have a big say in the matter are sometimes deliberately excluded from decision-making. In some cases, advisory committees comparable with the JCVI existed but were not consulted. In other countries EPI managers were not asked for their views. Some officials who were interviewed explained that in their country, lobbying by the pharmaceutical industry had played a crucial role.

Pressure from lobbyists, or the wish to get a share of international funding, are not the kind of justifications that parents want to hear, but there is little doubt that both play a role. Helen Burchett and her fellow researchers found that in Guatemala, EPI staff were asked to submit a funding request for rotavirus introduction in mid-2009. They declined, as they felt the programme was not ready for introduction of a new vaccine. In December 2009, they were told that the vaccine would be introduced anyway. Experts, and the normal consultation process, had been ignored. In poor countries, eligible for GAVI support, it seems that the availability of GAVI funding for rotavirus, or hepatitis B, or some other new vaccine, is itself sufficient to trigger an application – whatever the national priorities might previously have been. In other words, securing a share of GAVI funds may carry more political weight than actual health priorities, or consideration of the long-term implications of introducing a new vaccine. After all, the country is expected gradually to assume responsibility for the costs of the vaccine, especially once its national income rises above the GAVI threshold.

Introducing HPV

At the start of the millennium, more than half a million Americans died of cancer each year. Of the 273,000 American women who died of cancer in 2006, in 3,700 cases death was due to cancer of the cervix. This was far fewer than the 72,000 who died of lung cancer or the 41,000 who died of breast cancer, but obviously by no means negligible. Although in almost all cases cervical cancer is caused by a virus, the human papilloma virus (HPV), few women were aware of this at the time. Those who were probably knew that most sexually active women became infected by the virus at some point, though it very rarely caused any illness and generally cleared by itself. Moreover, where an illness was developing, in women who attended for regular screening (the PAP smear) this could generally be picked up and treated before it reached the cancerous stage.

For Merck, awaiting FDA approval of their new HPV vaccine, these perceptions did not suggest that there would be much demand. The fact that the price of the vaccine to the individual consumer would be something like $120 for each of the required three shots – far more than any existing vaccine – would not help. This was certainly a vaccine against a cancer, but since the virus is transmitted in the course of sexual intercourse it is also an STD. Trials had shown that the vaccine was likely to be most efficacious when given to girls, teens or pre-teens, before they became sexually active.

If their vaccine were to be a commercial success, Merck would have to create a market for it. In the USA they could utilize the mass, and later social, media to appeal directly to potential consumers. The initial purpose of the campaigns was not so much to market the vaccine, as to heighten attention to cervical cancer and to sensitize women to the fact that it was caused by a virus. The fact that this virus was transmitted through sexual intercourse was treated gingerly. Analysing Merck's campaigns, Laura Mamo and her colleagues explain how the company tried to avoid awkward and controversial questions of girls' sexuality.[17] The campaigns set out first to frame cervical cancer as a major public health concern, and then Merck's vaccine, Gardasil, as the best way of protecting against it. Despite the small number of deaths it caused, 'cervical cancer was transformed from a relatively rare cancer with an effective health-care infrastructure for prevention and early detection into a death sentence, a "disease of innocence", and a major public health concern.'[18] In other words, we see the same 'rebranding' that we came across with regard to mumps and measles. After the vaccine had been approved by the FDA, in June 2006, recommendations for its use in the United States quickly followed. It was to be offered to girls aged eleven to twelve, with women aged thirteen to 26 being eligible for a 'catch-up immunization'. The vaccine would be made available under the Vaccines for Children programme that President Clinton had established in 1993, so that girls from poor or Native American families would also have access to it. Advertising directed at young women, at women's groups and at physicians was stepped up. The manufacturer lobbied for HPV vaccination to be made compulsory: a move backed by the CDC and a number of other organizations active in the field of women's and reproductive health. Such 'mandates' would have to be introduced by the individual states. But this recommendation became highly controversial, provoking powerful opposition, not only from anti-vaccination groups, but also from libertarian groups and from the religious right, which saw it as an invitation to promiscuity.

In the UK, the JCVI initially recommended that all twelve- to thirteen-year-old girls be vaccinated, with a catch-up campaign for those aged fifteen to eighteen coming later. Instead of worrying about the uncertain duration of protection, as their German counterparts were doing, the JCVI made an 'educated guess' as to what it would be. Studies that were carried out showed that routine vaccination of girls aged twelve to fourteen years 'could reasonably be expected to be cost-effective at 80 per cent vaccine coverage, assuming the average duration of vaccine protection is at least 10 years'.[19] An initial uptake of 70–80 per cent was predicted. In 2007 the first empirical data relating to the UK itself came from a study carried out in Manchester. Three shots of the vaccine had been offered to nearly three thousand schoolgirls, and of these 70 per cent turned up for the first dose and slightly fewer for the second dose (though some of them only when the vaccination was rescheduled). Most of the parents who explained why they would not allow their daughters to have the vaccine said that too little was known of its effects. In September 2008 a national HPV vaccination programme began in the UK, aiming initially to provide three doses within the course of a school year.

No previous vaccine introduction had been accompanied by anything like the same level of public debate, though what exactly was being debated, and by whom, differed from country to country. In some countries, where manufacturers contributed visibly to debate, widespread awareness of their influence on politicians may have stimulated resistance to the vaccination. Medical associations and consumer advocacy groups played important, but varied, roles. For example, in Canada, New Zealand, Australia and the USA, most medical and public health agencies and societies supported a voluntary subsidized programme. In both Canada and New Zealand, women's health advocacy organizations either opposed the programme or expressed concerns about the speed of introduction and the lack of knowledge regarding long-term effects. The start of vaccination didn't end discussion. In France and Spain there have been recent court cases claiming damages. In 2011 the American conservative Republican presidential candidate Michele Bachmann was forced to back down from a claim she'd made that the vaccine caused brain damage.

In the course of the last few years, most European countries have started vaccinating against HPV. As of 2012 those that had not were largely the new EU member states in Central and Eastern Europe, where cervical cancer mortality is actually higher than in Western Europe. Austria is one of a handful of Western European countries that chose not to introduce the vaccine nationally (though it can be bought) because it did not seem cost-effective, but possibly also as a result of concern over safety. Andrea Stöckl, who studied its introduction in Austria, Germany and Italy, points out that the worries about encouraging promiscuity, which had played such an important role in the USA, were wholly absent from media discussions in these countries.[20]

Since the start of these programmes, various changes have been made. At the end of 2009, the FDA approved Gardasil for boys, to protect them against genital warts and cancer of the anus, and in 2011 the CDC recommended vaccination of boys aged eleven to twelve. In the UK the JCVI found that for girls vaccinated at under fifteen years of age, a two-dose schedule was effective, and in September 2014 the UK switched from a three-dose to a two-dose schedule. The vaccination of boys has aroused controversy in the UK, since the JCVI has said it is awaiting the results of a modelling exercise and will not recommend the vaccination of boys for the time being. In Japan, policy has moved in a different direction. In 2012, just after HPV vaccination started there, acceptance rates were comparable with those elsewhere. The government had recommended the vaccination of twelve-year-old girls, and Japanese parents tend to trust their government. Then, in June 2013, the recommendation was withdrawn, following reports of more than two thousand adverse events. The ministry of health did not suspend vaccination, but instructed local governments not to promote its use pending studies of adverse effects such as long-term pain and numbness. A study carried out in the city of Sakai, Osaka Prefecture, found that the effects were dramatic.[21] Girls in the seventh grade of school were expected to turn up for their vaccination during the summer vacation. During the summer vacation period in 2012, nearly half of them turned up, and overall more than 65 per cent were vaccinated. The next year hardly anyone turned up during the summer and the overall vaccination percentage fell to under 4 per cent.

The death rate from cervical cancer is far higher in the developing countries of Asia and Africa than it is in countries with well-developed health systems and well-organized screening programmes such as the UK or Japan. Compared to the four thousand cervical cancer deaths annually in the USA and thirteen thousand in the EU, there are something like 57,000 in the WHO's Africa region and 94,000 in the Southeast Asia region. In Africa, cancer mortality is well below mortality from infectious diseases, perinatal mortality and respiratory and diarrhoeal diseases. However, of the cancer-related causes of death in women, cervical cancer ranks highest, above breast cancer (unlike in Western Europe). Since these are countries in which few women have access to PAP screening, it seems clear that this is where the vaccine could do most good. Among the more than fifty countries eligible for GAVI support, cervical cancer is the leading cause of cancer deaths among women. The question for the organization and its sponsors was whether this vaccine could be effectively administered there, and the alliance has supported some 'demonstration projects' that it claims provide an answer in the affirmative.

As early as 2006 a United States-based NGO called PATH (Program for Appropriate Technology in Health), which works in seventy countries and has an annual budget of around $300 million, began a multi-year project in India, Peru, Uganda and Vietnam, which also addressed the question of feasibility. This was not supposed to be a clinical trial, but an exploration of practical feasibility – a distinction that would later be questioned. In 2011, GAVI added HPV to the list of vaccines it would support in poor countries, and it was able to negotiate a price of only $4.50 per dose, compared to the $130 per dose that an individual might pay in the USA. However, uncertainty has not been dispelled.

In 2009 PATH launched a study of HPV vaccination in the Indian states of Andhra Pradesh and Gujarat, in collaboration with the Indian Council of Medical Research (ICMR) and the state governments. Also described as a 'demonstration project', the study involved the vaccination of thirteen thousand girls aged ten to fourteen with Gardasil (in Andhra Pradesh) and ten thousand with Cervarix (in Gujarat). Controversy erupted a year later when a team of women's rights activists visited one of the study sites. Interviewing girls who had been vaccinated and health staff, they discovered that many trial participants were from particularly disadvantaged backgrounds and communities, that health infrastructures were 'woefully inadequate', and that large numbers of girls and their parents were simply unaware that they were part of a research project.[22] The women's rights activists concluded that the way in which the study had been conducted violated all relevant ethical guidelines. There had been no follow-up of four deaths believed to have been caused by the vaccination. Nor had the many side effects reported to the team of activists been either recorded or investigated. When the women's rights group released their report a public outcry followed.

Though the PATH study had been intended to run until 2011, in April 2010 the central government health minister announced a halt to all HPV vaccine trials in the country. Although an internal government inquiry exonerated the project, concluding that the deaths were unrelated to the vaccination and that no ethical guidelines had been breached, the Indian Parliament reached a different conclusion. The Parliamentary Standing Committee on Health and Family Welfare concluded that the study *had* violated India's laws and regulations. All its sponsors, PATH, the ICMR and the two state governments, were criticized. Despite the fact that it had been designated a 'demonstration project' (intended to explore how the vaccine could best be delivered and how to raise community awareness), the parliamentary committee concluded that it should in fact have fallen under clinical-trials legislation. Properly informed consent should have been obtained from all study participants (many of whom were illiterate), and adverse events should have been recorded and followed up.

Responding, PATH denied that this had been a clinical trial, since no clinical outcomes were measured. There is something odd here. If no clinical effects were being measured, and the study was not a clinical trial, then we can only assume that the value of the HPV vaccines in and for Indian populations had simply been taken for granted, based on the results of trials elsewhere. Reflecting on some of these events, critics raised a whole range of questions concerning the influence of multinational pharmaceutical companies, international organizations and foreign NGOs on the country's health policies and priorities. They question the rationality of introducing a vaccine that is unproven in India, and the cost of which is likely to draw resources from already inadequate screening services. 'The vaccine', they write, 'cannot be a substitute for comprehensive public health services.'[23] It is the causes of vulnerability, including the absence of healthcare, that need to be addressed. As of 2015, the matter was before the Supreme Court of India. When the central government recently announced that it nevertheless intended to add HPV to the country's Universal Immunization Programme, a letter protesting against the decision, signed by almost seventy representatives of public health and women's health organizations, and health researchers, was sent to the minister of health.

Taking Stock: The Free Trade Years

Public health has always been political, as Virchow pointed out long ago, and vaccination policies have always been subject to the vagaries of politics. We see this wherever we look, whether at the influence of

Cold War rivalries on polio vaccination in the two Germanys, or at resistance to the start of Clinton's Vaccines for Children programme in the U.S. Still, in the course of the past three decades, and corresponding more or less with the emergence of a new economic and ideological order in the 1980s, the logic underpinning vaccination policies has changed significantly.

All the vaccines introduced prior to that time offered protection against diseases that took many lives, generally those of children. Vaccination was to save lives, and it did. Not only the older vaccines against diphtheria, whooping cough and tetanus, but the new viral vaccines against polio and measles developed in the 1960s and '70s, saved millions of children's lives in the communities that had access to them. Because polio epidemics aroused such universal fear in temperate northern countries, an epidemic almost always led to the rapid start of a vaccination campaign. Measles vaccination began more gradually, though public health officials were generally convinced of its value. In the USA, an advertising campaign spearheaded by the vaccine's manufacturer set out to rebrand the disease as dangerous. In Western European countries, with their generally higher vaccination rates, policymakers were more concerned with whether parents would be willing to accept a vaccine against a disease they regarded as non-serious. If they were not, there was a fear that forcing it on them could undermine faith in the vaccination system as a whole. It was this that had to be avoided at all costs. There were also worries related to the duration of protection afforded by the vaccine, which was initially unknown. If the measles virus no longer found a breeding ground in immune children, might it find a new home in adults, in whom the consequences of infection would be more serious? Policymakers in the UK and other European countries wanted answers to these questions before recommending the start of universal vaccination, even when, as with measles, the value of vaccination was ultimately not in doubt.

In the case of mumps, the need for vaccination really was in doubt, even among physicians, in North America and in Western Europe. No one died of mumps, and though there were potential complications, these were relatively rare and could be cured with antibiotics. If mumps continued to be regarded as a mild disease, one of those temporary miseries that go with a normal childhood, there would be no market for Merck's new mumps vaccine. So we see the start of a strategy of 'rebranding', one that is now becoming ubiquitous. Through advertising and in other ways, American parents and their physicians were encouraged to fear mumps. As they learned to see it no longer as a normal part of childhood but as a potential source of neurological damage, demand for the vaccine followed. The fact that its manufacturer in the U.S., Merck, combined it with measles and rubella antigens made its introduction inevitable. In Europe, manufacturers were unable to use advertising to convince parents that their children should be protected against mumps. Nor would vaccine advisory committees have been swayed by advertising – even if it had been permitted. Mumps vaccination in the Netherlands began for two reasons. Taken together they illuminate the changing grounds on which decisions were being made. First, policymakers were convinced they could save on the costs of caring for sick children – though national data on which to base the calculation were not available. Data collected elsewhere would suffice. And second, neighbouring countries had begun to vaccinate against mumps and there was a growing conviction that European integration would require the country to harmonize its vaccination schedule with those of other countries. Of course, while these arguments might convince politicians to approve a new vaccine introduction, they would not convince many parents to bring their child to be given it. Even when there is a national vaccination programme for which no payment is required, parents still have to be convinced that mumps, or chickenpox, or a rotavirus infection, or a papilloma virus infection, is risky. A shift has taken place in the responsibilities of health policymakers. Widespread doubt, and the possibility that an unwelcome change in the vaccination schedule might undermine confidence in the vaccination programme as a whole, is no longer much of a reason for delaying. The obligation policymakers face today is no longer to listen to parents' doubts but to convince them that they have no reason to doubt. Parents must come to accept that what they had always thought a mere nuisance is in fact a serious illness.

Parents *have* to be convinced for a reason that derives from the increasing constraints on national action. At the national level, health policymakers are under all sorts of pressures to 'toe the line'. In the 1970s, as healthcare budgets came under pressure, cost–benefit and cost-effectiveness analyses became a welcome addition to the policymaker's armamentarium. Vaccination could easily be shown to be well worth the money. Today, though new vaccines are vastly more expensive than old ones, and the economic calculus is more complex, the idea that vaccination is a cost-effective tool of preventive health remains. Of course, it might be, and often it will be. But whether it is or not, and the answer will necessarily vary from country to country (though frequently the data do not exist so data from elsewhere must be used), the aura of cost-effectiveness is tightly attached. As a public health strategy it has a lot to commend it to anxious politicians trying to cope with inadequate budgets. At the same time, global health discourse is replete with vaccination coverage statistics, while global organizations such as GAVI praise countries that rapidly introduce a new vaccine and wag a finger in the direction of those that do not. Poor coverage, or failure to take advantage of a new vaccine (when neighbouring countries have done just that) is shaming. It has become very difficult, if not impossible, for a minister of health publicly to defend any kind of alternative health strategy in a global forum. These pressures are, of course, felt far more acutely in countries dependent on donor support for much of their health budget. While richer European countries can pursue an independent line for a while (not introducing chicken-pox vaccine, for example, or limiting hepatitis B vaccination to risk groups, or limiting HPV vaccination to girls only), pressures to con-form to the decisions of neighbouring countries and to conform to WHO guidelines, and pressure from the pharmaceutical industry, will eventually oblige them to toe the line.

Politicians face still greater pressure to keep in line when the objective is global eradication. However limited the resources and whatever health problems the country faces, it is this global objective which has to be prioritized. Despite Halfdan Mahler's warning years ago, the idea of disease eradication was enthusiastically adopted by a group of influential people, largely from the USA, and is being pushed vigorously, despite the fact that in the more poverty-stricken states, with the most fragile health systems, this might be at the cost of basic health services, including routine immunization. The Indian health activists who consistently question the way in which decisions to introduce new vaccines are taken are not alone in their sense that vaccine policy has moved further and further from any correspondence with the health needs of local communities. Crucial decisions are made in supranational organizations, the accountability of which is wholly unclear. Whoever's interests vaccination policy now reflects, whoever's healthcare concerns it now addresses, few people today can feel confident that it reflects their interests or addresses their concerns.

EIGHT

THE ROOTS OF DOUBT

Deep Roots

I n organizing this book I've discussed vaccines as particular kinds of
technologies. They are a set of tools that can be used for protecting the health of people and of communities: not the only tools for
doing so, but now crucially important ones. Like any tool, vaccines
can be used well or badly, appropriately or inappropriately. Scientific
discoveries, new insights, are put to use in searching for better tools,
for better ways of doing things. Innovators, developing a 'smart'
device, or a brain scanner, or a genetic test, are inspired by a particular problem or practice that they hope their new tool will address
better than anything else that's available. The history of technology
shows that quite commonly, as a new tool becomes widely available,
users seek and find other uses for it. Its production and use may
generate jobs, professional practices and new institutions. I used
the example of the car to suggest how a technology can come to
have a variety of meanings for people using it, or involved with it, in
different ways. Vaccines are no different, and it is absolutely crucial
not to lose sight of the distinction between the technologies on the
one hand, and the ways in which they are used on the other. Both the
development and production of vaccines, and the policies and practices through which they are put to use, have changed over time. And
though both have responded to the political, social and economic
upheavals of the past century, they have done so differently. They
have different histories. In this final chapter I am going to argue that
it is these changes, in the organization of vaccine production on the
one hand, and in vaccination policy on the other, that have given rise
to the loss of faith in vaccines and vaccination which has become
so widespread and which worries public health professionals. I am

going to suggest that providing parents with more and more detailed information on one vaccine or another is never going to solve the problem. Its roots lie elsewhere. Let me first briefly summarize the changes detailed in earlier chapters.

In the first half of the twentieth century, vaccines were developed and produced in public-sector institutes closely linked to departments of health, or in private companies that largely served local markets and were generally willing to collaborate with the public sector in a shared attack on infectious diseases. From the earliest days, the days of Jenner, Pasteur and Koch, the diseases that preoccupied vaccine scientists were those that killed and maimed. Even if research became skewed towards diseases that bothered the rich countries, the vaccines that emerged, for example against diphtheria, yellow fever, measles and whooping cough, were of great value to poor countries too. Then, in the ideological climate of the 1980s, things began to change. As scientists were exploring new ways of making vaccines, the skills and the knowledge involved, once shared in the interests of public health, were increasingly privatized. They were turned into 'intellectual property'. With the entry to the field of biotech companies with no history of public health involvement, and concerned principally with selling their expertise for the best possible return, the vaccine industry changed. In thrall to market economics, concerned by the rising costs both of healthcare and of vaccine development, politicians stripped their public health systems of the skills with which to respond to national health priorities. Vaccine development was best left to the pharmaceutical industry, even though it had not always been reliable in the past. Allowing free play to market forces came to seem the only way of doing almost everything. As 'shareholder value' was increasingly prioritized, and industry became increasingly oriented to profit maximization, interest in developing vaccines with limited market potential declined still further. Modern vaccines are sophisticated products embodying the most advanced science and technology, difficult and expensive to develop, and potentially very profitable. They have become a, if not *the*, principal source of growth in the pharmaceutical industry.

From a commercial perspective it obviously makes sense to develop any vaccine for which a profitable market can be established. Establishing that market, in the face of public indifference, may mean reframing a disease in the minds of public health policymakers or the population at large. The objective has to be to convince the world that if a vaccine can be made, it should be used: that any threat, or potential threat, that can in principle be reduced by vaccination is worth the effort. Why let your child run any risk at all? Healthcare in general is no longer limited to curing disease, as the rapid growth in 'lifestyle medicine' shows well enough. So, similarly, the scope of vaccination is being extended far beyond the prevention of life-threatening infectious diseases. Where once vaccine development took its priorities from what were clearly major threats to the health of the community, this is no longer wholly the case. There was never a need to persuade people to fear tuberculosis, cholera, polio or yellow fever. Popular perceptions of common conditions can be influenced, and we are made to fear illnesses that our parents used to view with a resigned shrug of the shoulders. What we see today is that increasingly well-informed populations are recognizing that new vaccines are an insufficient and not necessarily desirable response to the health challenges of our time.

If we now turn to the other side of the coin, to vaccination policy, the influence of political and economic changes, and of changes in the system of international relations, have been much greater. But the consequences for popular perceptions of vaccines and vaccination have resonated with those of changes in vaccine development.

Why is all that effort devoted to polio vaccination when the health system is so underfunded that it can't meet our basic needs? Concern at the decline of health services is no longer limited to African countries. Studies of materially deprived communities in the UK find that people living there have little trust in any of the institutions that they see as affecting their health and well-being. It is not limited to doctors and hospitals. There is resentment at the effects of cuts on health services in the community, but this resentment spills over:

> It soon became clear that [participants in the study] interpreted 'health' as a holistic issue and, therefore, directly associated it with other issues in their environment. It was also evident that local people felt disillusioned, socially excluded . . . and that they were relating their experiences and perceptions of health services to this more generalized feeling.[1]

Things have only got worse as austerity measures have cut deeper and deeper. With more and more people even in wealthy countries forced to rely on food banks and food stamps, unable to pay the rent or the interest on their mortgage, seeing no prospect of a decent job, there is a growing disillusionment with mainstream politics and politicians, and with states that seem unwilling or unable to stop the erosion of public services, the corruption of public institutions or the excesses of the financial sector.

In the 1970s, European health policymakers were cautious, far more cautious than their American counterparts, when it came to adding new antigens to the immunization schedule. This was partly, though not only, a matter of cost. In the United States measles vaccination was launched with the aid of an advertising campaign spearheaded by the vaccine's manufacturer. Western European policymakers moved more cautiously. They wanted to know whether parents would accept a vaccine against a disease that was widely regarded as non-serious. There was a fear that if parents were reluctant, forcing it on them could undermine faith in the vaccination system as a whole. It was this that had to be avoided at all costs. Though soon convinced that it was beneficial, policymakers in the UK and other European countries wanted to understand societal acceptability before introducing universal measles vaccination. Little room is allowed for such caution today. Widespread doubt, the possibility that an addition to the vaccination schedule might undermine confidence in the vaccination programme as a whole, is no longer a legitimate reason for delaying. The obligation policymakers face today is not to listen to parents' doubts but rather to argue them away.

Recall how even among physicians there was little sense that a mumps vaccine was needed. If everyone continued to think of mumps as a temporary misery that goes with a normal childhood, there would be no market for the new vaccine. So we see the start of the strategy of 'rebranding' that is now becoming ubiquitous. Through advertising and in other ways, American parents and their physicians were encouraged to fear mumps. As they learned to see it not as a normal part of childhood but as a potential source of neurological damage, demand for the vaccine grew. The fact that it was then combined with measles and rubella antigens made its introduction inevitable. The start of mumps vaccination in the

Netherlands had nothing to do with saving lives. It was because policymakers were convinced that they could save on the costs of caring for sick children, and because they were convinced that the moves to further European integration would require the harmonization of vaccination schedules. Of course, while arguments like these might convince politicians, they will not convince parents. Other arguments, public arguments invoking risk to a child's health, are needed if parents are to be convinced that mumps, or chickenpox, or a rotavirus infection, or a papilloma virus infection, is risky. If they are not convinced, not only will vaccination targets not be met, but confidence in the programme as a whole is jeopardized.

Parents *have* to be convinced because otherwise coverage will be low and the country will look bad in international comparisons. It is becoming more and more difficult for national representatives to get up in international gatherings and say, 'Well, we have other priorities.' They are under growing pressure to conform. When the EPI began in the 1970s, the international organizations involved, principally the WHO and UNICEF, were committed to assisting national governments in expanding their immunization programmes in ways that countries themselves considered most important. It was up to the individual countries to decide what their priorities were and which vaccines would be of greatest value to them. They would be helped with collecting the demographic and health-system data on which planning an expanded immunization programme could be based. As far as possible, immunization was to be integrated with other child-health services. It was the overall quality of healthcare that had to be optimized, and not so much vaccination coverage. Today health officials are under pressure to introduce new vaccines, whatever national needs or priorities might be, and irrespective of whether or not they even have the data on which to base an assessment of the burden of disease. In the case of a global eradication campaign, such as the polio campaign and its putative successors, the pressure is still greater. A global eradication programme, such as the GPEI, forces countries which may face major health problems to divert scarce manpower, funds and attention to something that is by no means their priority.

Vaccines are tools of public health to be used alongside other tools in protecting the health of populations, and children in particular. Decades ago there was little doubt as to which infectious diseases posed the biggest threat to children's health. Vaccines were acknowledged to be a 'technological fix', useful because tackling the root causes of these diseases was too difficult or too expensive. Today the means has become the end, with vaccine coverage as much as the burden of disease, let alone quality of life, having become the principal indicator of progress in the health field. Vaccination-coverage statistics are everywhere. GAVI's website is full of numbers: numbers of children who have been vaccinated against pneumococcus or meningitis, for example, and numbers still to be reached. Countries that have recently introduced a new antigen are signalled out for praise. Poor coverage, or failure to take advantage of a new vaccine, especially when neighbouring countries have done just that, is shaming. Obviously, as I pointed out earlier, countries dependent on international donors for a major share of the costs of running their health systems are necessarily the most responsive to pressures to conform. They can't look the proverbial gift horse in the mouth. Rich Western European countries have a little more leeway. They can choose not to introduce chickenpox vaccine, for example, or to limit hepatitis B vaccination to risk groups, or to offer HPV vaccine to girls only. For a while. Within just a few years, I suspect, pressures (to conform to neighbouring countries or to WHO guidelines, or from the pharmaceutical industry) will oblige them too to toe the line.

Overall, looking at the world as a whole, vaccine coverage is rising. But it is also clear that more and more parents in some of the world's wealthiest countries are not having their children vaccinated, or at least not wholly according to the recommended vaccination schedule. Public health officials are worried. If coverage rates continue to fall the benefits of herd immunity could be lost. This would increase the risk of more, and more serious, epidemics of diseases like measles or whooping cough. There is an obvious need to understand what is going on, and to determine what could be done to set things right again. In trying to make sense of it, it has been usual to make a distinction between the causes of low vaccination rates in developing countries and falling vaccination levels in developed ones. The former are assumed to be due to badly organized and inaccessible vaccination programmes. Studies have shown that vaccination services are often organized with little regard for the constraints under which poor people live, while arrogance and insensitivity on the part of professional staff may exacerbate the problem. In setting out to understand what is going on in the developed world, why vaccination rates are declining, factors of this kind are usually set aside. The problem, it is assumed, must have a behavioural cause. In other words, its roots must lie in the decisions that parents make, and thus in the information and the institutions that influence those decisions, and not in the organization or accessibility of health services.

Resisting Vaccination

As we saw earlier, resistance to vaccination is as old as mass vaccination itself. When smallpox vaccination campaigns began, in the nineteenth century, they often faced popular resistance. It was not just a matter of angry individuals refusing to get vaccinated. There were people who objected to the campaign as such and who organized themselves in order to make their views known. Their objection tended to be less to the *idea* of vaccination and more to the fact that it was being forced on people. Early in the twentieth century, the anti-vaccination movement declined, as health services improved and as laws in many countries were changed to allow people to opt out on grounds of conscience or religious beliefs.

Some commentators have seen continuities between the anti-vaccination movement of the late nineteenth century and present-day groups critical of vaccination. For example, comparing arguments used by the modern anti-vaccination movement with those used by its nineteenth-century counterparts, some authors find 'uncanny similarities, suggesting an unbroken transmission of core beliefs and attitudes'.[2] There is the suggestion that opposition to vaccination generally springs from deeply held beliefs of a spiritual or philosophical nature, and which have remained more or less unchanged for two centuries. Who are today's 'anti-vaccinationists', and are they indeed motivated by 'core beliefs and attitudes' unchanged from those of the nineteenth-century opponents of vaccination?

In the decades following the end of the Second World War, not all parents took for granted that vaccination was always in their child's interest. To be sure, objections to polio vaccination were rare. Serious epidemics, which had killed and maimed so many children, were still fresh in people's memories. Polio was frightening. Everyone had seen photos and newsreels of people lying in iron lungs, or of long lines of children waiting for their shot or vaccine-impregnated sugar cube. For most parents, protecting your child against polio was something you simply had to do. Objections to polio vaccination tended to come only from strongly religious communities, though in some countries, including the Netherlands, their views were respected and vaccination was never made mandatory. But in the industrialized world, measles and mumps were not really frightening, since almost all children caught them and recovered with no harm done. As we saw in earlier chapters, it took time and effort to convince parents that they should get their child vaccinated against what most of them regarded as fairly trivial childhood conditions. If a vaccination campaign were to succeed, parents would have to be convinced or cajoled, one way or another. In some places, a government recommendation was sufficient. In other places, departments of health resorted to public-relations campaigns and advertising techniques. But there was little or no organized opposition to vaccination in the industrialized world, and little or nothing was heard of the anti-vaccination arguments of the nineteenth century. But in the late 1970s vaccine critique re-emerged, and grew, and some vaccination rates began to fall. Public health doctors and politicians wanted to know what was going on. They needed an explanation.

Whooping cough vaccination was at the centre of it. A vaccine against whooping cough (pertussis) had been widely used since the 1950s, generally combined with diphtheria and tetanus toxoids in the DPT vaccine. Since its introduction, the incidence of whooping cough, which can be fatal in a small child, had fallen dramatically. But the whooping cough vaccine had side effects. Many children reacted badly to it and were obviously distressed after receiving their shot. Although side effects were, medically speaking, not serious, and generally disappeared within a day or two, they alarmed many parents. And by the late 1970s, when few young parents remembered pre-vaccine whooping cough epidemics, these side effects loomed large. Then rumours that the vaccine could cause brain damage began to circulate, seemingly backed by epidemiological research. In Sweden and in Britain, some doctors questioned the wisdom of vaccinating all babies against pertussis. In Sweden, Professor Justus Ström estimated that children receiving the full three doses of the vaccine ran a one in 170,000 chance of permanent brain damage.

In Britain, Gordon Stewart, professor of public health at Glasgow University, was similarly critical of the vaccine. His views sparked a controversy, which spilled over from medical journals into the daily press. In the late 1970s *The Guardian* covered it at length. Parents claiming compensation for the damage they believed the whooping cough vaccine had caused established an Association of Parents of Vaccine Damaged Children. Questions were asked in Parliament, and in 1979 the British government introduced a Vaccine Damage Payment Act, on the grounds that if the state recommended vaccination the state should be responsible in the event of injury. A similar controversy arose in Japan, leading to a national debate regarding vaccine-related adverse events. In each of these countries, confidence in pertussis vaccine declined dramatically throughout the 1970s and so, as a result, did vaccination coverage. This was especially marked in Sweden and in Japan, where coverage fell from 80–90 per cent to around 10 per cent. In the United States, public concern over the vaccine led to hundreds of lawsuits, claiming billions of dollars in damages. Fearful of crippling litigation, all but two U.S. manufacturers of DPT withdrew from the market, provoking fears of vaccine shortage. This was a major incentive for the establishment, in 1986, of the National Childhood Vaccine Injury Compensation Program, designed to reassure parents, but above all to reassure the vaccine manufacturers.

The vital thing for public health authorities was to restore public confidence in the vaccination programme as a whole. In Britain the Ministry of Health resisted pressure to withdraw the vaccine, and was able to reassure people sufficiently. Gradually, the coverage rate rose again. However, both Swedish and Japanese authorities suspended pertussis vaccination. In both countries experts had decided that a new and safer whooping cough vaccine was required, and that the existing vaccine should no longer be used. It was in this context that Japanese scientists began to study how to develop a different vaccine that would not cause these side effects. Building on their work, vaccine manufacturers responded with a new, so-called 'acellular', pertussis vaccine, from which the surface proteins that caused the side effects had been removed.

In the 1970s the controversy that had caused British and Swedish pertussis vaccination rates to plummet did not affect the Netherlands, where Stewart's work, though known, aroused no controversy whatsoever. There were references to British studies reporting brain damage in the principal Dutch medical journal, but no one thought it worth carrying out a similar study in the Netherlands. Throughout the whole of the decade, neither the daily press nor popular women's magazines carried any warnings of possible risks of brain damage as a result of pertussis vaccination. Whether because of very different responses from the media in the two countries, or because of medical consensus in the Netherlands, or the prompt action of the State Institute of Public Health (RIV) in investigating the single reported case of possible brain damage (which was found to be due to other causes), the Netherlands avoided the controversy. There was no decline in public confidence in the vaccine and no decline in vaccination coverage, and there were no demands for compensation payments.

In Britain, although confidence in the pertussis vaccine was eventually restored, by the 1990s attitudes to vaccination had nevertheless changed. An indication of growing popular concern is the fact that newspapers were devoting more and more space to vaccination. One study found a huge increase in the number of published articles on vaccine-related topics through the 1990s, but also an increase in the share of articles that dealt specifically with vaccine safety.[3] What is more, it was precisely at this time, the 1990s, that organizations critical of vaccination began to re-emerge. Most were established by parents demanding more complete, or less one-sided, information; or the right to choose which vaccines their child should receive; or easier access to compensation in the event of something going wrong as a result of vaccination. In Britain, The Informed Parent was established in 1992, principally to promote freedom of choice with regard to vaccination. In support of this objective it provided information on vaccines and it encouraged parents to consider alternatives to vaccination. In 1994 John and Jackie Fletcher set up Justice, Awareness and Basic Support (JABS). Convinced their child's health had been damaged by the MMR vaccine, the Fletchers contacted other parents who felt the same way. JABS presented itself specifically as a support group for vaccine-damaged children, with 'recognition' and 'compensation' as its principal objectives. Claims for compensation for damage alleged to have been caused by MMR, being pursued through the British courts, were a major issue for JABS. Yet another group in the UK was the Vaccine Awareness

Network, founded in 1997 by two parents who were dissatisfied with the quality and availability of vaccine information. Its website explains that its objective is 'to enable parents to make a fully informed choice about their child's vaccinations'.

Although the whooping cough controversy had not affected the Netherlands in the 1970s, there too a vaccine-critical association, the Nederlandse Vereniging Kritisch Prikken (NVKP), was established in 1994. Some of its founders were parents, while others had become critical as a result of their professional experience. Finding that few practitioners of orthodox medicine gave them satisfying answers to the questions they had, they set up the NVKP.

The chances are that few people today remember the 1970s pertussis vaccine controversy. It has been displaced by a more recent and somewhat comparable controversy around the MMR vaccine. In February 1998, Andrew Wakefield, at the time a gastroenterologist working in London, published a paper in *The Lancet*, together with twelve co-authors, in which the MMR vaccine was suggested to have caused autism and bowel disease in children. The paper was based on a very small sample without controls, and pretty soon it attracted criticism on methodological grounds. That was only the start of a long-running saga that led to the paper's being retracted by the journal twelve years later, after journalist Brian Deer appeared to have shown its results to be fraudulent and the General Medical Council had decided that the research had been conducted unethically.[4]

In 2011 the editors of the *British Medical Journal* pointed out that while Wakefield had been given ample opportunity either to replicate the paper's findings or to admit to having made a mistake, he had refused to do either. Nor, in 2004, had he been willing to join ten of his co-authors in retracting the paper: 'Although now disgraced and stripped of his clinical and academic credentials, he continues to push his views.'[5] 'Meanwhile', the editorial goes on, 'the damage to public health continues, fuelled by unbalanced media reporting and an ineffective response from government, researchers, journals, and the medical profession.' Despite the scores of studies that disprove the link between MMR and autism, there are clearly still people, perhaps many people, who have not been convinced.

And Andrew Wakefield is far from forgotten. Now living in the United States, in August 2016 he is reported to have met with (then) presidential candidate Donald Trump.[6]

In March 2016 a film that almost no one had (or has) seen occasioned a brief uproar. Directed by Wakefield, the film is called *Vaxxed: From Cover-up to Catastrophe*. On 26 March the *New York Times* carried an article headed 'Tribeca Film Festival to Screen an Anti-vaccination Movie'. Director of this prestigious festival is the actor Robert De Niro, who is the father of a child with autism. De Niro initially defended his decision to show the film as facilitating open discussion around the supposed link between the MMR vaccine and autism, an issue important to him and his family. According to reports, the film consists largely of interviews with Wakefield himself and with a man called William Thompson, supposedly a CDC whistleblower, who claims that the CDC fudged the numbers to show that MMR vaccine was safe. Two days after defending inclusion of the film, De Niro issued a statement saying that he had decided to withdraw it from the festival after all. There were sighs of relief. On 29 March, *The Guardian* carried an article with the headline 'How the Scientific Community United against Tribeca's Anti-vaccination Film'. As soon as the screening of the anti-vaccine documentary *Vaxxed* was announced at Robert De Niro's festival, experts joined forces to oppose it.' In it, the newspaper's chief U.S.-based reporter, Ed Pilkington, goes on to explain how, as soon as the showing of the film became known, 'a well-oiled network of scientists, autism experts, vaccine advocacy groups, film-makers and sponsors cranked into gear to oppose it'.[7] As newspapers guessed they would, the angry filmmakers accused the festival organization of censorship, presenting withdrawal of the film as a free-speech issue.

The fact is that, until recently, a single explanation of declining vaccination rates has dominated the medical and public health press. The problem, everyone seemed to agree, was due to the activities of an anti-vaccination movement that had somehow re-emerged, and which liked to regard Andrew Wakefield as a persecuted hero. Modern anti-vaccination organizations like JABS and the NVKP are now armed with far more powerful ways of spreading their message than had been available to their nineteenth-century predecessors. No one thought to ask why these groups critical of vaccination had emerged *when* they did.

Thus, two medical scientists associated with the Mayo Clinic's vaccine-research group explain that the anti-vaccination movement (which they call an 'anti-vaccine' movement – which is not the same thing) has 'resulted in major disruptions and even cessation of vaccine programs, with resultant increased morbidity and mortality'. 'In measurable ways', they argue, 'the anti-vaccine movement has impacted state and national public health policy, and jeopardized individual and societal health.'[8] This view was widely shared in the public health community. Publications making a similar point have been very widely cited in the professional literature.[9]

The modern anti-vaccination movement is so dangerous, the explanation went, because it has ways of spreading its message that its predecessor could not have imagined: 'Anti-vaccine groups have taken advantage not only of the internet to increase their presence in the debate, but also to exaggerate, publicize and dramaticize [*sic*] cases of vaccine reactions to the media and the public.'[10] The traditional media, burdened by a pervasive ignorance of science, and eager to court sensation, also have to bear their share of the responsibility.

Public health professionals were worried that, seeking information, parents would most likely stumble on anti-vaccination websites. What exactly might they find there? Well, many of them claimed that adverse reactions to vaccination are under-reported; that vaccines cause idiopathic illness such as autism or diabetes; and that vaccine policy is shaped by drug companies looking for profit. There are still many such websites, claiming that vaccines are biological poisons, full of noxious additives such as antifreeze and formaldehyde, and are responsible for a variety of idiopathic illnesses including, of course, autism.[11] Many raise the question of parents' rights, which are said to be infringed when parents are not allowed to make their own choices regarding their child's health. Vaccination-related issues are now emerging in social media too. Though there is no actual evidence as to their effects on real-world behaviour,

> An analysis of YouTube immunization videos found that 32 per cent opposed vaccination, and that these had higher ratings and more views than pro-vaccine videos; 45 per cent of negative videos conveyed information contradicting reference standards. A YouTube analysis specific to HPV immunization . . . found that 25.3 per cent of videos portrayed vaccination negatively.[12]

An Easy Target

Attributing declining vaccination rates to misinformation spread through the Internet by misguided people has a feature that makes it particularly attractive in the world of international public health. To point an accusing finger at groups promoting junk science is to attribute responsibility to an identifiable culprit. Anti-vaccination groups are an enemy that can be outmanoeuvred or debunked. Since they mainly exist online, steps can be taken to ensure that search engines put official pro-vaccine sites first. Not that this was – or is – the only tactic being used. In Australia, in particular, critics of vaccination are subject to a campaign of vilification and intimidation. Sociologist Brian Martin, a professor at the University of Wollongong, has been following the campaign. The target is the Australian Vaccination Network (AVN), set up in 1994 by a woman called Meryl Dorey. Martin explains that it's pretty much like similar vaccine-critical groups elsewhere. It has a website, some two thousand member–subscribers and had, until recently, a magazine. The difference from similar groups elsewhere is the nature of the opposition it has faced. Brian Martin has described the activities of an organization, 'Stop the Australian Vaccination Network', or SAVN, established in 2009 by people hostile to alternative medicine and radically pro-vaccine. Its stated objective is to force the AVN to close down its website, to stop publication of its magazine, and to discourage media coverage of AVN or its leading members. Martin explains how SAVN first claimed (on its Facebook page) that the AVN 'believes in a global conspiracy to implant mind control chips via vaccination'. This curious accusation was later watered down. 'Secondly, SAVNers have made numerous derogatory online comments about the AVN and about AVN members who post public comments, especially Dorey. . . . Thirdly, SAVNers and others have made numerous formal complaints about the AVN to government agencies.'[13] Subsequently Brian Martin himself became the subject of attack.

Blaming organizations like Dorey's diverts attention from less tractable problems. It obscures the possibility that resistance to vaccination may somehow reflect failings in the way vaccination programmes work, or still more fundamental anxieties. Whatever its appeal, empirical research shows that blaming everything on anti-vaccination organizations doesn't hold up as an explanation. Studies that go beyond simply making assumptions about motivations, and give parents the opportunity of speaking for themselves, show that something much more complicated is involved. The Internet is not the sole, and is often not the most important, source of influence on parents' thinking about vaccination. Since making up their minds about the vaccination of their child can be quite difficult for many parents, they turn to friends, family and neighbours, as well as their medical practitioner, for information.

A study based on focus groups carried out with parents in Britain in 2001, when the MMR scare was fresh in people's minds, found that

> all parents felt that the decision about MMR was difficult and stressful, and experienced unwelcome pressure from health professionals to comply. Parents were not convinced by Department of Health reassurances that MMR was the safest and best option for their children and many had accepted MMR unwillingly.[14]

Nor were medical professionals all convinced. Interviews found British GPs and health visitors uncomfortable with the fact that the information they were given to pass on to parents was so obviously one-sided. Nor was patient trust helped by the fact that GPs were known to receive additional payments from the NHS if they reached immunization targets.

A study conducted a few years later in Brighton, an affluent university town on the English south coast, found that attitudes to vaccination were shaped by personal and family medical histories. Out of these mothers distilled a sense of their own children's vulnerabilities. Reflecting on the MMR vaccination, these mothers didn't think about it in the abstract. They thought about how it might affect their own child. And they wanted to take personal responsibility for their child's well-being, rather than leaving it to the state. One of these mothers, who was also a nurse, explained that she wasn't against the MMR vaccine in principle. The problem for her was that she felt there were uncertainties regarding its safety. When judgements regarding an individual child have to be made, then, in her view it is the child's parents who should make them:

I just think there should be a choice for parent to, you know, so that you can make the decision yourself. Unless something comes out that there is absolutely no link with autism, it is completely safe, I think the choice element should be there and that's how I felt at the time that I wanted to make that choice and that's what I chose for my children. But I just think the choice should be there for all parents.[15]

The value of a study like this, carried out in a distinctive locality, is that it shows how people's views about vaccination are not purely individual. Because people exchange views with friends and neighbours, particular ways of thinking about vaccination tend to predominate in particular communities. This has led some researchers to speak of 'local vaccine cultures'. Some of the details disclosed by this particular study may therefore be specific to the locality, Brighton, in which the study was conducted. However, researchers talking to parents in very different places have found similar sentiments expressed. In one recent study, carried out in Quebec (Canada), researchers interviewed women some weeks before and some weeks after the birth of their child. These mothers generally thought the 'old vaccines' safe and valuable, but were far less sure about new vaccines, such as the varicella or rotavirus vaccines.[16] Looking back, many mothers who'd vaccinated their child were not confident that they had made the right decision. A study in Brazil found something similar. Interviews with a sample of educated middle-class parents in São Paulo found that their doubts about vaccination had nothing to do with MMR. Their doubts were a symptom of something far more complex, which no amount of information on vaccine safety could possibly assuage. Their doubts reflect a loss of trust, and a much more diffuse sense of dissatisfaction with increasingly technological and dehumanized medical practice: precisely the concerns that are leading to the increasing popularity of complementary and alternative medicine in much of the world. These Brazilian women are adopting a selective approach to vaccination. As one put it,

With some new vaccines, we try to learn a bit more about them to see if they are worth it or not. But for the main ones, we vaccinate. The most dangerous diseases and the most traditional ones, we vaccinate and follow the vaccination card. It's the newer ones that we study more in depth. We listen to his [the paediatrician's] opinion, and do not provide some vaccines.[17]

Earlier, I quoted from the book in which Eula Biss, an American university teacher, describes how she began to think about immunization during her own pregnancy. She explains how her world, a world of educated professionals, is indeed riddled with doubts, anxieties and mistrust. Decisions, whether to immunize the child or not, are imbued with doubts and uncertainties much like those expressed by the Brazilian and French-Canadian parents interviewed in these studies. In other words, there is now evidence from various parts of the world that many parents, especially educated middle-class parents, are no longer willing to take vaccination recommendations on trust. The parents who actually refuse to vaccinate their children are the tip of an iceberg. Doubt is far more widespread, even among the majority of parents who do still accept all the recommended vaccines at the recommended times.

'Vaccine Hesitancy' and Vaccine Confidence

In the last few years there has been a somewhat half-hearted acknowledgement that thinking in black-and-white terms, in terms of a simple distinction between 'vaccine acceptance' and 'vaccine refusal', won't do. It fails to capture the uncertainties with which many parents seem to be struggling, whether they finally decide for or against vaccination. Whereas a decade ago 'vaccine refusal', which could readily be blamed on the anti-vaccinationists, was seen as the problem, in the last few years the public health community has started to focus on what is becoming known as 'vaccine hesitancy'.

In 2009 the WHO's vaccine advisory group, SAGE, noted that the attempt to eliminate measles in Europe was hampered by all sorts of problems, including 'a lack of political and societal support for the goal, propaganda by anti-vaccine groups, contrary religious and philosophical beliefs, competing health priorities, and problems created by the reform of health systems in some eastern European countries'.[18] Apparently unconscious of the irony involved in lumping 'lack of political and social support for the goal' together with 'propaganda by anti-vaccine groups', the conclusion was that the WHO's European region needed a new and more pro-active strategy for responding to anti-immunization activities.

This 'review of vaccine hesitancy' notes that in 2010 the European region was asked 'to use the European immunization week as a platform for increasing public awareness of the benefits of immunization and countering the false messages disseminated by anti-vaccination movements'. There is still a real reluctance, or perhaps an inability, to let go of the idea that it is all the fault of an anti-vaccination movement. Pronouncements remain ambiguous because entrenched ways of thinking could not, and perhaps cannot, get to grips with so slippery and intangible a phenomenon. In January 2010, a 'project to monitor public confidence in immunisation' was established.[19] The idea behind it was that with the help of a global network of informants, and by monitoring the Internet and social media, it should be possible to obtain a view of emerging vaccination-related public concerns. In other words, the project set out to apply the digital methods that epidemiologists now use to track emerging disease outbreaks through peaks in messaging. This new digital epidemiology is based on the perception that, long before official statistics have been collected and analysed, an epidemic outbreak will lead to people in the affected area increasingly communicating about it through digital media. The idea behind this project was that similar methods could be used to track emerging concerns relating to specific vaccines or immunization programmes. That is, the spread of vaccine-critical views or rumours would be mapped, through time and geographically, by using data extracted from social media.

In 2012, SAGE established a Working Group on Vaccine Hesitancy, which was to define the concept, develop indicators for measuring it and advise SAGE on how the problem could best be tackled.[20] Since the literature contained no established definition, there was prolonged discussion of whether 'hesitancy', with obviously negative connotations, was the best term to use. Might not 'confidence' be better? The working group decided to stick with 'vaccine hesitancy', which they defined as referring to 'delay in acceptance or refusal of vaccination despite availability of vaccination services. Vaccine hesitancy is complex and context specific, varying across time, place and vaccines. It is influenced by factors such as complacency, convenience and confidence.'[21] In other words, what is at issue is being clearly distinguished from situations in which low uptake is due to parents lacking information or facing financial or other barriers to accessing vaccination services. The focus of concern should be the educated middle-class urban parents who hesitate because they are not wholly convinced of the benefits of vaccination, and who may ultimately decide not to vaccinate their children. The concept is being adopted with growing enthusiasm. Not only is it finding its way into more and more scholarly publications, but influential figures in the public health world are stressing that it needs to be studied with care. For example, in an editorial in the prestigious journal *Science*, Barry Bloom, one-time dean of the Harvard School of Public Health, and co-authors emphasized a need for 'research that addresses how and when attitudes and beliefs about vaccines are formed, how people make decisions about immunization, how best to present information about vaccines to hesitant parents, and how to identify communities at risk of vaccine-preventable disease outbreaks'.[22]

This and most other writing on the subject shows how far the concept of vaccine hesitancy embodies core assumptions taken over from the world-view of the public health profession. Personally I believe that these assumptions will actually block any real understanding of what is involved. The vaccination experts who meet in SAGE ask for a *clear definition* of vaccine hesitancy with the aid of which the phenomenon can be *measured*. A problem with working with a clear definition, as I pointed out earlier, is that it assumes away the diversity of potentially conflicting meanings surrounding an artefact, practice or belief. This variety of meanings could be crucial, as might the different ways in which they interact with practical and material constraints on vaccination. There is also an assumption that beliefs about vaccination are *stable* ('how and when they are formed'), though I doubt that this is so. Trying to make something fixed and measurable comes at a price. Even when authors are clearly well aware that 'vaccine hesitancy' has complex roots, they seem to be at a loss to do anything other than bring their established tools to bear on what they know and can measure (in effect, rates of non-vaccination). For example, in a recent article entitled 'Epidemiology of Vaccine Hesitancy in the United States', researchers from the schools of public health at two leading universities show themselves to be very aware of the complexity of the issue.[23] They point to a decline of trust in the large pharmaceutical companies that make vaccines and in the government that promotes them. They point to widespread anxiety regarding relationships between industry, the medical profession and government. They point to parents no longer wanting to be told what to do for their children's health. All of these 'sociocultural changes have contributed to vaccine hesitancy'. Yet by the end of the article, 'vaccine hesitancy' has somehow turned into 'vaccine refusal'. It is this, vaccine refusal, that poses a risk both to individual children and to communities, and which needs to be tackled. 'Increased efforts are required to improve and maintain public confidence in vaccines', especially 'evidence based interventions'.[24] The implication is that the solution can be found, and the problem solved, using the tools of epidemiology and public health. Personally I do not believe that this is so. Here is an example that I think supports my case.

In much of the world, recent HPV vaccination campaigns have failed to elicit the expected popular response. It was soon quite clear that this was not due to anti-vaccination propaganda on the Internet. Still less could the decision of the Japanese government, in 2013, to withdraw its recommendation that all twelve-year-old girls be vaccinated be explained in that way. There was a clear need to probe more deeply, and many studies of HPV uptake have been carried out, principally in the United States but also in European countries. Worldwide figures on HPV vaccination coverage show considerable differences between countries.

Norway is at one extreme. When voluntary HPV vaccination was introduced for girls in their early teens, 78 per cent turned up for the first shot. Of these, more than 95 per cent (74 per cent of all the girls) completed the full three shots. Studying the statistics, researchers found some variation between groups, but differences were very small. Girls with mothers older than age fifty at the time of their daughter's scheduled vaccination were slightly less likely to turn up compared to girls with younger mothers. HPV vaccine initiation was a bit higher among girls whose mothers had the lowest education, and lower for girls whose mothers had the highest education. Norway, of course, has a rather cohesive population, a tradition of egalitarianism, and a more highly developed welfare state than most countries. Few countries can match Norway's vaccination coverage rate. Thus compared to the 74 per cent of Norwegian girls who had had the full three shots, only 39 per cent of German girls had done so. Or compare Norway with the United States. In the USA, in 2014, 60 per cent of thirteen- to seventeen-year-old girls had received one dose, but less than 40 per cent had received all three. Moreover, inter-group variation was vastly greater than in Norway, though studies come to conflicting conclusions regarding the nature of this variation. Some studies find vaccination coverage to be lower among Caucasian girls, while other studies find it to be higher, compared with girls from ethnic minorities, among whom cervical cancer is more common. Even when they have ready access to healthcare, which many did not, young African American women are less likely to be vaccinated against HPV than their Caucasian peers. A study of a small Asian minority, girls of Cambodian origin, found that scarcely any had completed the full schedule. While 33 per cent of girls aged thirteen to seventeen had received one shot, only 14 per cent had received all three.[25] Although there is no simple explanation for this, it suggests to me that the categorical separation between material restrictions on vaccination and behavioural 'hesitancy', assumed to be independent of each other, is misleading. In a world of increasing inequality, economic marginalization and cultural marginalization are likely to reinforce one another.

In the United States researchers have devoted a lot of attention to studying class and ethnic variation in HPV uptake. However, as I pointed out earlier, the kind of correlations they typically look for offer little insight into how differences arise. Knowing that girls from one ethnic group are more likely to be vaccinated than girls from another may suggest where health workers and information campaigns need to focus their efforts. But it does not say much about what underlies such differences. Epidemiological studies of inter-group variance in HPV vaccine uptake throw very little light on the differences in sexual practices, or in attitudes to risk, or in religious beliefs, or trust in official institutions, that lie behind the numbers. Nor can they tell us anything about how girls are influenced by the stories circulating in schools or in online communities.

Even when authors claim to be addressing 'vaccine hesitancy' rather than 'vaccine refusal', they still seem to assume that people's doubts about vaccines and vaccinations can be dealt with without delving into the tangled roots of the problem. It is not difficult to see why epidemiologists and public health doctors prefer not to have to think about popular mistrust of the pharmaceutical industry or its influence on the medical profession. But the question is whether the problem that concerns them can be analysed, let alone tackled, without doing so.

I think the answer is that it cannot, so that current analyses will be unable to get to grips with growing vaccine-related doubts and anxieties.

Vaccination Resonances

Although organized resistance to vaccination had more or less disappeared from Western countries by the 1930s, this was not true everywhere. Earlier I said a little about the BCG vaccination campaign that began soon after the end of the Second World War and which was extended to India in 1948. The campaign encountered significant resistance in the newly independent country, and for two distinctive sorts of reasons. For the national government, the appeal of the vaccination campaign was that it offered a feasible and effective way of dealing with the tuberculosis that was ravaging the country. Those who objected, many of them based in Madras (now Chennai), denied that a health problem so clearly bound up with the country's widespread poverty could be solved by a single technological solution. From the government's perspective, dealing with the root causes, the poverty and living conditions of the country's vast population, was simply not feasible. This tension, between tackling root causes as against using available technologies to deal with the worst symptoms, was of course translated to the international level in the subsequent controversy around universal or selective primary healthcare.

But the analysis shows that something else, at least as fundamental, was also at stake. That 'something else' was no less than the values that the struggle for Indian independence had expressed, and the kind of country India was to become. The fact that the BCG campaign involved using outside knowledge, applied by foreign experts, to solve an indigenous problem fitted ill with powerful nationalist post-colonial sentiments. India had its own medical traditions, which many preferred. The Madras-based leader of the resistance chose to attack the BCG campaign because a more powerful symbol of Nehru's modernist pretensions would have been hard to find. The immunization plan was a scheme devised largely by outsiders and the central government, which would require Indians to submit to a medical practice that many found objectionable.[26]

It would be a mistake to dismiss these events as of interest only to historians because they took place in India more than half a century ago. Their importance here is that they show how a vaccination campaign can be invested with symbolic importance. It can come to stand for the institutions promoting it, and can act as a focus for wider disaffections. Parents make connections with other things that the state has done to them or for them, or to ways in which it has failed them. Thus, in a study carried out in Uganda in the 1990s, Harriet Birungi found that attitudes to injections provided by government health centres had changed as a result of deterioration in the country's health system. Starting in the 1970s, when the dictatorship of Idi Amin led to economic breakdown, government resources for healthcare had declined. Scant resources did not allow for proper supervision or for health workers to be paid a living wage. Immunization programmes scarcely functioned. Birungi explains that continuing economic failure meant that medical professionals survived by ignoring their normal professional ethics, for example starting to demand under-the-counter payments for services that were officially free, or misappropriating drugs and equipment for private practice. This breakdown in service provision, coupled with widespread departure from professionally ethical practice, led to an erosion of trust in state healthcare institutions and in professional knowledge.[27] A vaccination campaign can also act as a conduit for collective memory; for memories of state oppression, ethnic conflicts, or past injustice. Little wonder that rumours regularly attach themselves to such campaigns, or that anthropologists have studied them.[28]

Vaccination-related rumours rarely provoke much of a furore in public health circles, even when described by anthropologists in scholarly journals. But in the context of a global eradication campaign, disruptive rumours can acquire a totally different significance, as shown by events in northern Nigeria a decade ago. In 2003, religious leaders in parts of northern Nigeria, which is predominantly Muslim, became convinced that the oral polio vaccine in use there had been deliberately contaminated with anti-fertility drugs and AIDS-inducing agents. A number of northern Nigerian states then banned use of the vaccine, and polio vaccination there stopped. In the midst of the global eradication programme this horrified the international health community and attracted a good deal of critical attention in Western media. It was taken for granted that the problem was due to superstition, ignorance or something similar and, in line with earlier assumptions about anti-vaccinationism, could be solved by providing the facts. The federal government arranged tests of the vaccine, which showed that it was not contaminated, but to no avail. Northerners were unwilling to be convinced. As Nigerian scholars later pointed out, the issue was actually about more than just the safety of the vaccine. It was tied up with a variety of anxieties, memories and discontents: with memories of colonialism and with the region's post-colonial history. The country's internal politics also played a role, in particular the ongoing post-independence struggle between the country's main ethnic groups over political power and autonomy. Northern Nigerians mistrusted a federal government that had recently come under southern domination:

> To sum up, the polio vaccination crisis as a whole provides a paradigm of emergent tensions between the North and the South that are best understood in light of historical relations between the two. . . . It also clearly shows up the deepening immersion of health in the domain of politics, coupled with the increasingly political nature of health issues in the contemporary world.[29]

In Nigeria mistrust was fuelled by a widespread feeling that the further erosion of already inadequate primary healthcare was due to federal government policy. People simply could not understand why this one disease was receiving such disproportionate resources, when most people could not even afford basic medicines to treat minor ailments. Northern Nigerians had reasons for doubting that the national and international agencies responsible for the polio programme had their best interests at heart. The polio vaccine was made to symbolize their disaffection. When asked, people in other countries express similar concerns. Anthropologists have found that wherever large numbers of parents have refused vaccination, whether it is in Africa or in South Asia, similar issues crop up in interviews. Asked why they had not taken their child to be vaccinated against polio, parents refer to a mismatch between the well-funded polio eradication programme and a health system unable to meet their most basic healthcare needs. It makes people angry, and it leads them to question the motives behind the polio vaccination programme.

Resistance may also represent the crystallization of resentments slowly simmering, perhaps for decades, ignited by injustices of the past. Though most accounts of broader dissatisfactions being projected onto vaccination programmes come from the Global South, it is not a uniquely Southern phenomenon. In Europe, too, attitudes to state vaccination programmes can become infused with memories of past injustices, as Cristina Pop's study of HPV vaccination in Romania shows so beautifully.[30] Pop explains how the government planned to provide the vaccine, free, through school medical services. This was in 2009, just twenty years after the corrupt authoritarian regime of Nicolai Ceauşescu had been brought down. Parents would have to give their permission, but so few did so that after two months only 2.5 per cent of the target population had been vaccinated. The programme was suspended and relaunched a year later. Pop shows how, in explaining why they had withheld consent, many parents and grandparents evoked a deep-rooted mistrust of state healthcare, and indeed of the Romanian state in general. She explains that they 'were linking apparently disconnected topics (such as mistrust in state-provided reproductive care, apprehensions regarding additive-laden foods, radioactivity, and environmental pollution, and praise for maternal milk) in their HPV vaccination refusal narratives, under broader themes of purity and corruption.' There were fears that the state was covertly seeking to regain the control over the private lives of its citizens that it had had under the previous regime.

The sentiments that influence parents and that help shape their attitudes to vaccination, may go far beyond anything to do with the risk of infectious disease, or confidence in the safety of a particular vaccine. They may be of a religious character, and to that extent it does make sense to think of beliefs shared with some of the anti-vaccination protestors of the nineteenth century. They may be associated with a preference for holistic healthcare, and here too it makes sense to think of continuities with objections inspired by earlier holistic health movements. But what events like these, in Nigeria, Romania and Uganda, show is that confidence in the state, and in the services it provides, is always potentially infused with memories of what the state has done in the past. Various lessons might have been drawn from studies like these, showing how a state vaccination programme can come to stand for government policies and priorities more generally, and can serve as a focus for resistance to those policies. The public health profession is reluctant to draw lessons like these since their implications are so challenging, and go so far beyond its own professional competences.

Vaccine hesitancy is fuelled by awareness that the vaccination policies to which people are expected to conform are being formulated not by their elected representatives but in hazy supranational organizations, the accountability of which is wholly unclear. People know this and have become mistrustful. It is also fuelled by attitudes to the pharmaceutical industry, which, as a recent survey in the UK found, are overwhelmingly negative.[31]

Sometimes mistrust is amplified by broader resonances, through which vaccines, vaccination and the vaccinator are seen as 'standing for' the institutions (the state, the medical profession, technoscience) on which they rest. Refusing vaccination might then be one of the small acts of rebellion by which people with little power often express their discontents.

To end, then, much of the explanation of 'vaccine hesitancy' is to be found in the field of vaccination itself, though not in the sense that it can be measured or resolved with the traditional tools of public health. To understand it, we have to look at the vaccines field as a whole, and specifically at the changes in its structure that I have tried to document in this book. As vaccines became increasingly vital both to international public health and to the pharmaceutical industry, a tension emerged between their function in public health and their profitability as high-tech commodities. Vaccines have saved countless lives and, suitably deployed, can save countless more. But believing this, as I do, does not commit me to a belief in the universal benefit of all vaccines that industry might see fit to produce. It makes no sense to say 'I'm pro-vaccine' or 'I'm anti-vaccine'. What I hope the analysis in this book has shown is the complexity of what lies behind declining confidence in vaccination programmes – the phenomenon that is coming to be known as 'vaccine hesitancy'.

To be sure, this is a problem *for* public health, but in my view it is neither resolvable nor even adequately analysable with the tools or the concepts *of* public health. Rudolf Virchow's famous claim that politics is nothing but medicine writ large – that is to say that public health cannot but be political – has been set aside. Still, I am convinced that defining, measuring, mapping – the tools of epidemiology – will shed little light on a phenomenon rooted in the lack of trust which now infects public and political life more generally. Specifically, a community's acceptance or rejection of a vaccination programme reflects its trust in the institutions responsible for that programme. In recent decades, as vaccines have acquired increasing commercial importance for companies competing in a global market, these institutions have become more and more obscure, less and less responsive to people's own perceptions of threats to children's health. A consequence has been that trust and accountability have declined in tandem.

REFERENCES

1 WHAT DO VACCINES DO?

1 Charles E. Rosenberg, *Explaining Epidemics and Other Studies in the History of Medicine* (Cambridge, 1992).
2 Ibid., p. 287.
3 Roy Porter, 'Plague and Panic', *New Society* (12 December 1986), p. 11.
4 Nathan Wolfe, *The Viral Storm: The Dawn of a New Pandemic Age* (London, 2011), p. 98.
5 Ibid., p. 242.
6 J. E. Suk and J. C. Semenza, 'Future Infectious Disease Threats to Europe', *American Journal of Public Health*, CI/11 (2011), pp. 2068–79.
7 National Institutes of Health (NIH), *Understanding Vaccines*, www.violinet.org/docs/undvacc.pdf.
8 MSF (Doctors without Borders), 'The Right Shot: Bringing Down Barriers to Affordable and Adapted Vaccines', 2nd edn (2015); available at www.msfaccess.org.
9 Veena Das, 'Public Good, Ethics, and Everyday Life: Beyond the Boundaries of Bioethics', *Daedalus*, CXXVIII/4 (1999), pp. 99–133.
10 Ibid.
11 Paul Greenough, 'Intimidation, Coercion and Resistance in the Final Stages of the South Asian Smallpox Eradication Campaign, 1973–1975', *Social Science & Medicine*, XLI/5 (1995), pp. 633–45.
12 Eula Biss, *On Immunity: An Inoculation* (Minneapolis, MN, 2014), pp. 20–21.
13 Ibid., p. 24.
14 Richard Krause, 'The Swine Flu Episode and the Fog of Epidemics', *Emerging Infectious Diseases*, XII/1 (2006), p. 42.
15 Peter Baldwin, *Contagion and the State in Europe, 1830–1930* (Cambridge, 2005).
16 *The Compact Edition of the Oxford English Dictionary* (London, 1979), p. 3581. Reprint of the 1971 edition published by Oxford University Press.
17 H. J. Parish, *A History of Immunization* (Edinburgh and London, 1965).
18 Porter, 'Plague and Panic'.
19 Nadja Durbach, *Bodily Matters: The Anti-vaccination Movement in England, 1853–1907* (Durham, NC, and London, 2005).
20 *The Compact Edition of the Oxford English Dictionary*, p. 3581.

2 TECHNOLOGIES: THE FIRST VACCINES

1 Friedrich Engels, *Condition of the Working Class in England* (New York and London, 1891); available at www.marxists.org.
2 Edwin Chadwick, *Report on the Sanitary Condition of the Labouring Population of Great Britain* (London, 1842), republished with an introduction by Michael W. Flinn (Edinburgh, 1965).
3 Ibid., pp. 2–73.
4 René Dubos and Jean Dubos, *The White Plague: Tuberculosis, Man and Society* (New Brunswick, NJ, 1992), p. 46.
5 Ibid., p. 65.
6 Ibid., p. 99.
7 Jonathan M. Liebenau, 'Public Health and the Production and Use of Diphtheria Antitoxin in Philadelphia', *Bulletin of the History of Medicine*, LXI/2 (1987), p. 235.
8 Volker Hess, 'The Administrative Stabilization of Vaccines: Regulating the Diphtheria Antitoxin in France and Germany, 1894–1900', *Science in Context*, XXI/2 (2008), pp. 201–27.

3 TECHNOLOGIES: VIRAL CHALLENGES

1 Frederick C. Robbins, 'Reminiscences of a Virologist', in T. M. Daniel and F. C. Robbins, *Polio* (Rochester, NY, 1997), pp. 121–34.
2 Aaron E. Kline, *Trial by Fury: The Polio Vaccine Controversy* (New York, 1972), p. 110.
3 Centre for Disease Control and Prevention, 'Report of Special Advisory Committee on Oral Poliomyelitis Vaccines', *Journal of the American Medical Association*, CXC/1 (1964), pp. 161–3.
4 Hans Cohen, quoted in Stuart Blume and Ingrid Geesink, 'Vaccinology: An Industrial Science?', *Science as Culture*, IX (2000), p. 60.
5 Office of Technology Assessment (OTA), *A Review of Selected Federal Vaccine and Immunization Policies* (Washington, DC, 1979).

4 TECHNOLOGIES: THE COMMODIFICATION OF VACCINES

1 Institute of Medicine (IOM), *New Vaccine Development: Establishing Priorities* (Washington, DC, 1986).
2 Jon Cohen, 'Bumps on the Vaccine Road', *Science*, 265 (September 1994), pp. 1371–5.
3 Ruth Nussenzweig, quoted ibid., p. 1371.
4 Phyllis Freeman and Anthony Robbins, 'The Elusive Promise of Vaccines', *American Prospect*, IV (1991), pp. 8–90.
5 William Muraskin, *The War against Hepatitis B: A History of the International Task Force on Hepatitis B Immunization* (Philadelphia, PA, 1995), p. 27.
6 Freeman and Robbins, 'The Elusive Promise', p. 84.

7 Louis Galambos with Jane Sewell, *Networks of Innovation: Vaccine Development at Merck, Sharp and Dohme and Mulford 1895–1995* (Cambridge, 1995).

8 National Centre for Disease Control, 'Quarterly Newsletter of the National Centre for Disease Control', III/1 (2014), pp. 1–4; available at www.ncdc.gov.in.

9 Craig Wheeler and Seth Berkeley, 'Initial Lessons from Public–private Partnerships in Drug and Vaccine Development', *Bulletin of the World Health Organization*, LXXIX (2001), p. 732.

10 *The Economist* Data Team, 'Ebola in Africa: The End of a Tragedy?', www.economist.com, 14 January 2016.

11 M. Kaddar, 'Global Vaccine Market Features and Trends', World Health Organization (Geneva, 2013); available at http://who.int/influenza_vaccines_plan/resources/session_10_kaddar.pdf.

5 POLICIES: HESITANT BEGINNINGS

1 James Colgrove, *State of Immunity: The Politics of Immunization in Twentieth-century America* (Berkeley, CA, 2006), p. 334.

2 Ibid., p. 96.

3 René Dubos and Jean Dubos, *The White Plague: Tuberculosis, Man and Society* (New Brunswick, NJ, 1992), p. 712.

4 Ibid., p. 176.

5 Linda Bryder, '"We Shall Not Find Salvation in Inoculation": BCG vaccination in Scandinavia, Britain and the USA, 1921–1960', *Social Science & Medicine*, XLIX (1999), pp. 1157–67.

6 POLICIES: VACCINATION AND THE COLD WAR

1 Dora Vargha, 'Between East and West: Polio Vaccination across the Iron Curtain in Cold War Hungary', *Bulletin of the History of Medicine*, 88 (2014), p. 334.

2 I am grateful to Maria Fernanda Olarte-Sierra for the following anecdote that shows the durability of the assumption that 'the poor' are carriers of disease: 'When we worked on dengue in Villavicencio (Colombia) the whole campaign was based on the rhetoric of the "poor". Villavicencio has a huge socio-economic gap between the "rich" and the "poor". Given that healthcare workers went house-by-house talking about prevention of this "disease of the poor", people living in well-off areas considered this information irrelevant and would call their maids, drivers, nannies, etc. to hear the information, since *they* were "the poor" . . . When looking at breeding sites, houses of rich people had small fountains, which proved to be a fantastic breeding place for the mosquitoes . . . but they did not . . . take any of the necessary precautions and were falling sick with dengue. They assumed that their servants were infecting them.' See M. Roberto Suarez, Maria Fernanda Olarte-Sierra et al., 'Is What I Have Just a

Cold or is it Dengue? Addressing the Gap between the Politics of
Dengue Control and Daily Life in Villavicencio-Colombia', *Social
Science & Medicine*, LXI (2005), pp. 495–502.
3 Quoted in Socrates Litsios, 'The Long and Difficult Road to Alma-Ata:
A Personal Reflection', *International Journal of Health Services*, XXXII/4
(2002), pp. 709–32.
4 Julia Walsh and Kenneth Warren, 'Selective Primary Health Care:
An Interim Strategy for Disease Control in Developing Countries',
New England Journal of Medicine, CCCI (1979), pp. 967–74.
5 Alexander Langmuir, D. A. Henderson, R. E. Serfling and I. L. Sherman,
'The Importance of Measles as a Health Problem', *American Journal
of Public Health*, LII (1962), p. 3.
6 World Health Organization, 'Consultation on the WHO Expanded
Programme on Immunization', report of a meeting held in Geneva,
30 April–3 May 1974 (WHO file 18/87/2).
7 Resolutions of the 27th World Health Assembly, Resolution WHA 27.57,
Geneva, 23 May 1974.
8 Dr Alfa Cissé, speech at the 29th World Health Assembly, Geneva,
May 1976. Document A29/A/SR15, p. 11.
9 Ann Mills, 'Vertical Versus Horizontal Health Programmes in Africa:
Idealism, Pragmatism, Resources and Efficiency', *Social Science &
Medicine*, XVII (1983), p. 1977.
10 Dr A. Geller, address to a seminar organized by the WHO Regional
Office for Africa, Brazzaville, October 1976. Document AFR/CD/51.
11 R. H. Henderson, 'The Expanded Program on Immunization of
the World Health Organization', *Reviews of Infectious Diseases*, VI,
Supplement 2 (1984), p. S477.
12 Kenneth Newell, 'Selective Primary Health Care: The Counter
Revolution', *Social Science & Medicine*, XXVI (1988), p. 905.
13 S. Gloyd, J. Suarez Torres and M. A. Mercer, 'Immunization
Campaigns and Political Agendas: Retrospective from Ecuador and
El Salvador', *International Journal of Health Services*, XXXIII/1 (2003),
pp. 113–28.
14 Anne-Emanuelle Birn, 'Small(pox) Success?', *Ciencia & Saude Coletiva*,
XVI (2011), pp. 591–7.

7 POLICIES: VACCINATION IN A GLOBALIZING WORLD

1 D. Walker, H. Carter and I. Jones, 'Measles, Mumps, and Rubella:
The Need for a Change in Immunisation Policy', *British Medical
Journal*, CCXCII/6534 (1986), pp. 1501–2.
2 N. S. Galbraith, S. E. Young, J. J. Pusey et al., 'Mumps Surveillance in
England and Wales 1962–1981', *The Lancet*, I/8368 (1984), pp. 91–4.
3 'Mumps Vaccination', *The Lancet*, CCXCIII/7609 (1969), p. 1302.
4 'Prevention of Mumps', *British Medical Journal*, CCLXXXI/6251 (1980),
p. 1231.
5 Elena Conis, *Vaccine Nation: America's Changing Relationship with
Immunization* (Chicago, IL, 2015).

6 Ibid., p. 82

7 Nancy Leys Stepan, *Eradication: Ridding the World of Diseases Forever?* (London, 2011).

8 William Muraskin, *Polio Eradication and Its Discontents* (New Delhi, 2012).

9 D. R. Hopkins, A. R. Hinman, J. P. Koplan et al., 'The Case for Global Measles Eradication', *The Lancet*, 1/8286 (1982), pp. 1396–8.

10 A. R. Hinman, W. H. Foege, C. de Quadros et al., 'The Case for Global Eradication of Poliomyelitis', *Bulletin of the World Health Organization*, LXV/6 (1987), pp. 835–40.

11 Ibid.

12 World Health Assembly, 'Global Eradication of Poliomyelitis by the Year 2000', WHA Resolution, WHA 41.28, World Health Organization, Geneva, 1988.

13 Svea Closser, *Chasing Polio in Pakistan* (Nashville, TN, 2010).

14 Isao Arita, Miyuki Nakane and Frank Fenner, 'Is Polio Eradication Realistic?', *Science*, 312 (2006), pp. 852–4.

15 Center for Disease Control and Prevention, 'Measles Eradication: Recommendations from a Meeting Cosponsored by the World Health Organization, the Pan American Health Organization, and CDC', *Mortality and Morbidity Weekly Report*, 46 (13 June 1997).

16 H.E.D. Burchett, S. Mounier-Jack, U. K. Griffiths et al., 'New Vaccine Adoption: Qualitative Study of National Decision-making Processes in Seven Low- and Middle-income Countries', *Health Policy & Planning*, XXVII (2012), supplement 2, pp. ii5–ii16.

17 Laura Mamo, Amber Nelson and Aleia Clark, 'Producing and Protecting Risky Girlhoods', in *Three Shots at Prevention: The HPV Vaccine and the Politics of Medicine's Simple Solutions*, ed. K. Wailoo, J. Livingston, S. Epstein and R. Aronowitz (Baltimore, MD, 2010), pp. 121–45.

18 Ibid., p. 127.

19 L. Brabin, S. A. Roberts, R. Stretch et al., 'Uptake of First Two Doses of Human Papilloma Vaccine by Adolescent Schoolgirls in Manchester: Prospective Cohort Study', *British Medical Journal*, CCCVI (2008), pp. 1056–8.

20 Andrea Stöckl, 'Public Discourses and Policymaking: The HPV Vaccination from the European Perspective', in Wailoo et al., *Three Shots*, pp. 254–70.

21 Yutaka Ueda, T. Enomoto, M. Sekine et al., 'Japan's Failure to Vaccinate Girls against Human Papilloma Virus', *American Journal of Obstetrics & Gynecology*, 212 (2015), p. 405.

22 N. B. Sarojini , S. Srinivasan, Y. Madhavi et al., 'The HPV Vaccine: Science, Ethics and Regulation', *Economic & Political Weekly*, XLV/48 (2010), pp. 27–34.

23 Ibid., p. 33.

8 THE ROOTS OF DOUBT

1 Paul Ward and Anna Coates, 'We Shed Tears, but There Is No One There to Wipe Them Up for Us: Narratives of (Mis)trust in a Materially Deprived Community', *Health*, x (2006), pp. 283–301.

2 R. M. Wolfe and L. K. Sharp, 'Anti-vaccinationists Past and Present', *British Medical Journal*, CCCXXV (2002), p. 430.

3 C. Cookson, 'Benefit and Risk of Vaccination as Seen by the General Public and Media', *Vaccine*, XX (2002), S85–S88.

4 Brian Deer, 'How the Case against the MMR Vaccine was Fixed', *British Medical Journal*, CCCXLII (2011), pp. 77–82.

5 Fiona Godlee, Jane Smith and Harvey Markovitch, 'Wakefield's Article Linking MMR Vaccine and Autism was Fraudulent', *British Medical Journal*, CCCXLII (2011), p. 65.

6 Z. Kopplin, 'Trump Met with Prominent Anti-vaccine Activists during Campaign', *Science* (November 2016); available at www.sciencemag.org.

7 Ed Pilkington, 'How the Scientific Community United against Tribeca's Anti-vaccination Film', *The Guardian* (29 March 2016), www.theguardian.com.

8 G. A. Poland and R. M. Jacobson, 'Understanding Those Who Do Not Understand: A Brief Review of the Anti-vaccine Movement', *Vaccine*, XIX/17–19 (2001), p. 2441.

9 E. J. Gangarosa, A. M. Galazka, C. R. Wolfe et al., 'Impact of Anti-vaccine Movements on Pertussis Control: The Untold Story', *The Lancet*, CCCLI/9099 (1998), pp. 356–61.

10 Poland and Jacobson, 'Understanding', p. 2442.

11 Anna Kata, 'A Postmodern Pandora's Box: Anti-vaccination Misinformation on the Internet', *Vaccine*, 28 (2010), pp. 1709–16; Anna Kata, 'Anti-vaccine Activists, Web 2.0, and the Postmodern Paradigm: An Overview of Tactics and Tropes Used Online by the Anti-vaccination Movement', *Vaccine*, XXX (2012), pp. 3778–89.

12 Kata, 'Anti-vaccine Activists', p. 3779.

13 Brian Martin, 'Censorship and Free Speech in Scientific Controversies', *Science & Public Policy*, XLII (2015), pp. 377–86.

14 M. Evans, H. Stoddart, L. Condon et al., 'Parents' Perspectives on the MMR Immunisation: A Focus Group Study', *British Journal of General Practice*, LI (2001), pp. 904–10.

15 M. Poltoraka, M. Leach, J. Fairhead and J. Cassell, '"MMR Talk" and Vaccination Choices: An Ethnographic Study in Brighton', *Social Science & Medicine*, LXI (2005), p. 717.

16 Eve Dubé, Maryline Vivion, Chantal Sauvageau et al., '"Nature Does Things Well, Why Should We Interfere?" Vaccine Hesitancy Among Mothers', *Qualitative Health Research*, XXVI/3 (2016), pp. 411–25.

17 Carolina Alves Barbieri and Marcia Couto, 'Decision-making on Childhood Vaccination by Highly Educated Parents', *Revista Saúde Pública*, XLIX/18 (2015), pp. 1–8.

18 Heidi J Larson, David M. D. Smith and Pauline Paterson, 'Measuring Vaccine Confidence: Analysis of Data Obtained by a Media

Surveillance System used to Analyse Public Concerns about Vaccines', *Lancet Infectious Diseases*, 13 (2013) pp. 606–13.

19 Melanie Schuster, Juhani Eskola, Philippe Duclos, SAGE Working Group on Vaccine Hesitancy, 'Review of Vaccine Hesitancy: Rationale, Remit and Methods', *Vaccine*, XXXIII (2015), p. 4158.

20 N. E. MacDonald and the SAGE Working Group on Vaccine Hesitancy, 'Vaccine Hesitancy: Definition, Scope and Determinants', *Vaccine*, XXXIII (2015), pp. 4161–4.

21 Ibid.

22 B. R. Bloom, E. Marcuse, S. Mnookin et al., 'Addressing Vaccine Hesitancy', *Science*, CCCXLIV/6182 (2014), p. 339.

23 M. Siddiqui, D. Salmon and S. Omer, 'Epidemiology of Vaccine Hesitancy in the United States', *Human Vaccines and Immunotherapeutics*, IX (2013), pp. 2643–8.

24 Ibid.

25 V. M. Taylor, N. Burke, L. K. Ko et al., 'Understanding HPV Vaccine Uptake among Cambodian American Girls', *Journal of Community Health*, XXXIX/5 (2014), pp. 857–62.

26 Christian McMillen and Niels Brimnes, 'Medical Modernization and Medical Nationalism: Resistance to Mass Tuberculosis Vaccination in Postcolonial India, 1948–1955', *Comparative Studies in Society and History*, LII/1 (2010), p. 198.

27 Harriet Birungi, 'Injections and Self-help: Risk and Trust in Ugandan Health Care', *Social Science & Medicine*, XLVII/10 (1998), pp. 1455–62.

28 P. Feldman-Savelsberg, F. T. Ndonko and B. Schmidt-Ehry, 'Vaccines or the Politics of the Womb: Retrospective Study of a Rumor in Cameroon', *Medical Anthropology Quarterly*, XIV/2 (2000), pp. 159–79.

29 E. Obadare, 'A Crisis of Trust: History, Politics, Religion and the Polio Controversy in Northern Nigeria', *Patterns of Prejudice*, XXXIX (2005), p. 278.

30 Cristina Pop, 'Locating Purity within Corruption Rumors: Narratives of HPV Vaccination Refusal in a Peri-urban Community of Southern Romania', *Medical Anthropology Quarterly*, DOI: 10.1111/maq.12290.

31 YouGov Report, 'British Attitudes to the Pharmaceutical Industry', www.yougov.co.uk (30 August 2013).

ADDITIONAL READING

GENERAL

Bornside, George H., 'Waldemar Haffkine's Cholera Vaccine and the Ferran–Haffkine Priority Dispute', *Journal of the History of Medicine and Allied Sciences*, XXXIV (1982), pp. 399–422

Cueto, Marcos, ed., *Missionaries of Science: The Rockefeller Foundation and Latin America* (Bloomington, IN, 1994)

Delaporte, François, *Disease & Civilization: The Cholera in Paris, 1832*, trans. A. Goldhammer (Cambridge, MA, 1986)

Gauri, V., and P. Khaleghian, 'Immunization in Developing Countries: Its Political and Organizational Determinants', *World Development*, XXX (2002), pp. 2109–32

Harrison, Mark, *Contagion: How Commerce Has Spread Disease* (New Haven, CT, and London, 2012)

King, Nicholas B., 'Security, Disease, Commerce: Ideologies of Postcolonial Global Health', *Social Studies of Science*, XXXII (2002), pp. 763–89

Kraut, Alan M., *Silent Travellers: Germs, Genes, and the 'Immigrant Menace'* (New York, 1994)

Kumar, Sunil, *Decolonizing International Health: India and Southeast Asia, 1930–65* (London and New York, 1998)

Moreno, Jonathan D., ed., *In the Wake of Terror: Medicine and Morality in a Time of Crisis* (Cambridge, MA, 2003)

Moulin, Ann-Marie, 'The International Network of the Pasteur Institute, Scientific Innovations and French Tropisms', in *The Emergence of Transnational Intellectual Networks and the Cultural Logic of Nations*, ed. C. Charle, J. Schriewer and P. Wagner (New York, 2004), pp. 135–62

Nichter, Mark, 'Vaccinations in the Third World: A Consideration of Community Demand', *Social Science & Medicine*, XLI (1995), pp. 617–32

Offit, Paul A., *Vaccinated: One Man's Quest to Defeat the World's Deadliest Diseases* (New York, 2007)

Plotkin, Stanley, and Bernadino Fantini, eds, *Vaccinia, Vaccination, Vaccinology: Jenner, Pasteur and their Successors* (Paris, 1996)

Roalkvam, Sidsel, Desmond McNeill and Stuart Blume, eds, *Protecting the World's Children: Immunisation Policies and Practices* (Oxford, 2013)

Rosenberg, Charles E., *The Cholera Years: The United States in 1832, 1849, 1866* (Chicago, IL, 1962)

Streefland, Pieter, A. Chowdhury and P. Ramos-Jimenez, 'Patterns of
     Vaccine Acceptance', *Social Science & Medicine*, XLIX (1999), pp. 1705–16
Suarez, M. Roberto, Maria Fernanda Olarte et al., 'Is What I Have Just a
     Cold or Is It Dengue? Addressing the Gap between the Politics of
     Dengue Control and Daily Life in Villavicencio-Colombia', *Social
     Science & Medicine*, LXI (2005), pp. 495–502
Szreter, Simon, 'Industrialization and Health', *British Medical Bulletin*, LXIX
     (2004), pp. 75–86
Wills, Christopher, *Plagues: Their Origin, History and Future* (London, 1996)
World Health Organization, *Global Vaccine Action Plan, 2011–2020*,
     www.who.int/immunization

BACTERIOLOGY AND VIROLOGY

Amsterdamska, Olga, 'Medical and Biological Constraints: Early Research
     on Variation in Bacteriology', *Social Studies of Science*, XVII (1987),
     pp. 657–87
Geison, Gerald L., *The Private Science of Louis Pasteur* (Princeton, NJ, 1995)
Gradmann, Christoph, *Laboratory Disease: Robert Koch's Medical Bacteriology*
     (Baltimore, MD, 2009)
Löwy, Ilana, 'On Hybridizations, Networks and New Disciplines:
     The Pasteur Institute and the Development of Microbiology in
     France', *Studies in the History and Philosophy of Science*, XXV (1994),
     pp. 655–88
Waterson, A. P., and Lise Wilkinson, *An Introduction to the History of
     Virology* (Cambridge, 1978)

VACCINE INSTITUTIONS AND MECHANISMS

Cassier, Maurice, 'Producing, Controlling, and Stabilizing Pasteur's
     Anthrax Vaccine: Creating a New Industry and a Health Market',
     Science in Context, XXI (2008), pp. 253–78
Hilleman, Maurice, 'Vaccines in Historic Evolution and Perspective:
     A Narrative of Vaccine Discoveries', *Vaccine*, XVIII (2000),
     pp. 1436–47
Institute of Medicine, *America's Vital Interest in Global Health: Protecting
     Our People, Enhancing Our Economy, and Advancing Our International
     Interests* (Washington, DC, 1997)
Jadhav, Suresh, M. Datla, H. Kreeftenberg and J. Hendriks, 'The Developing
     Countries Vaccine Manufacturers' Network (DCVMN) is a Critical
     Constituency to Ensure Access to Vaccines in Developing Countries',
     Vaccine, XXVI (2008), pp. 1611–15
Liebenau, Jonathan, *Medical Science and Medical Industry: The Formation of
     the American Pharmaceutical Industry* (London, 1987)
Milstien, Julie B., P. Gaulé and M. Kaddar, 'Access to Vaccine Technologies
     in Developing Countries: Brazil and India', *Vaccine*, XXV (2007),
     pp. 7610–19

Mowery, David C., and Violaine Mitchell, 'Improving the Reliability of the
    U.S. Vaccine Supply: An Evaluation of Alternatives', *Journal of Health
    Policy Politics and Law*, XX (1995), pp. 973–1000
Muraskin, William, 'The Global Alliance for Vaccines and Immunization:
    Is it a New Model for Effective Public–private Cooperation in
    International Health?', *American Journal of Public Health*, XCIV (2004),
    pp. 1922–5
——, *The Politics of International Health: The Children's Vaccine Initiative and
    the Struggle to Develop Vaccines for the Third World* (New York, 1998)
Sandberg, Kristin, S. Andresen and G. Bjune, 'A New Approach to Global
    Health Institutions? A Case Study of New Vaccine Introduction and
    the Formation of the GAVI Alliance', *Social Science & Medicine*, LXXI
    (2010), pp. 1349–56
Weindling, Paul, ed., *International Health Organisations and Movements,
    1918–1939* (Cambridge, 1995)
——, 'Public Health and Political Stabilisation: The Rockefeller Foundation
    in Central and Eastern Europe between the two World Wars', *Minerva*,
    XXXI (1993), pp. 253–67

VACCINATION ATTITUDES AND OPPOSITION

Blume, Stuart, 'Anti-vaccination Movements and Their Interpretations',
    Social Science & Medicine, LXII (2006), pp. 628–42
Hobson-West, Pru, '"Trusting Blindly Can Be the Biggest Risk of All":
    Organised Resistance to Childhood Vaccination in the UK',
    Sociology of Health & Illness, XXIX (2007), pp. 198–215
Leach, Melissa, and James Fairhead, *Vaccine Anxieties: Global Science, Child
    Health & Society* (London, 2007)
Offit, Paul A., *Autism's False Prophets: Bad Science, Risky Medicine, and the
    Search for a Cure* (New York, 2008)
Ward, Jeremy K., 'Rethinking the Anti-vaccine Movement Concept: A Case
    Study of Public Criticism of the Swine Flu Vaccine's Safety in France',
    Social Science & Medicine, CLIX (2016), pp. 48–57
Yaqub, Ohid, S. Castle-Clarke, N. Sevdalis and J. Chataway, 'Attitudes to
    Vaccination: A Critical Review', *Social Science & Medicine*, CXII (2014),
    pp. 1–11

DIPHTHERIA

Hooker, Claire, and Alison Bashford, 'Diphtheria and Australian Public
    Health: Bacteriology and Its Complex Applications *c.* 1890–1930',
    Medical History, XLVI (2002), pp. 41–64
Hüntelmann, Axel C., 'Diphtheria Serum and Serotherapy: Development,
    Production and Regulation in Fin de Siècle Germany', *Dynamis*, XXVII
    (2007), pp. 107–31
Klöppel, Ulrike, 'Enacting Cultural Boundaries in French and German
    Diphtheria Serum Research', *Science in Context*, XXI (2008), pp. 161–80

Lewis, Jane, 'The Prevention of Diphtheria in Canada and Britain 1914–45', *Journal of Social History*, xx (1986), pp. 163–76

EMERGING INFECTIOUS DISEASES

Berkelman, Ruth, and Phyllis Freeman, 'Emerging Infections and the CDC Response', in *Emerging Illnesses & Society*, ed. R. M. Packard, P. J. Brown, R. L. Berkelman and H. Frumkin (Baltimore, MD, 2004), pp. 350–87

Fidler, David P., SARS, *Governance and the Globalization of Disease* (London and New York, 2004)

Garrett, Laurie, *The Coming Plague: Newly Emerging Diseases in a World out of Balance* (New York, 1994)

Hayes, Edward B., 'Zika Virus outside Africa', *Emerging Infectious Diseases*, xv/9 (2009), pp. 1347–50

Pennington, Hugh, 'Biting Habits', *London Review of Books* (18 February 2016), pp. 19–20

HEPATITIS B

Conis, Elena, '"Do we Really Need Hepatitis B on the Second Day of Life?" Vaccination Mandates and Shifting Representations of Hepatitis B', *Journal of Medical Humanities*, xxxii (2011) pp. 155–66

Madhavi, Yennapu, 'Manufacture of Consent? Hepatitis B Vaccination', *Economic and Political Weekly* (14 June 2003), pp. 2417–24

Millman, Irving, T. K. Eisenstein and B. S. Blumberg, eds, *Hepatitis B: The Virus, the Disease, the Vaccine* (New York, 1984)

Muraskin, William, 'The Silent Epidemic: The Social, Ethical, and Medical Problems Surrounding the Fight against Hepatitis B', *Journal of Social History*, xxii (1988), pp. 277–98

Stanton, Jennifer, 'What Shapes Vaccine Policy? The Case of Hepatitis B in the UK', *Social History of Medicine*, vii (1994), pp. 427–46

HIV/AIDS

Barnett, Tony, and Alan Whiteside, AIDS *in the Twenty-first Century: Disease and Globalization*, 2nd edn (London, 2006)

Cohen, Jon, *Shots in the Dark: The Wayward Search for an AIDS Vaccine* (London and New York, 2001)

Craddock, Susan, 'Market Incentives, Human Lives, and AIDS Vaccines', *Social Science & Medicine*, lxiv (2007), pp. 1042–56

Olin, John, J. Kokolamami, B. Lepira, K. Mwandagalirwa et al., 'Community Preparedness for HIV Vaccine Trials in the Democratic Republic of Congo', *Culture, Health & Sexuality*, viii (2006), pp. 529–44

Rhodes, Scott D., *Innovations in HIV Prevention Research and Practice through Community Engagement* (New York, 2014)

HUMAN PAPILLOMA VIRUS

Fernandez, Maria, E. J. Allen, R. Mistry and J. A. Kahn, 'Integrating Clinical, Community, and Policy Perspectives on Human Papillomavirus Vaccination', *Annual Reviews of Public Health*, XXXI (2010), pp. 235–52

Haas, Marion, T. Ashton, K. Blum et al., 'Drugs, Sex, Money and Power: An HPV Vaccine Case Study', *Health Policy*, XCII (2009), pp. 288–95

Mishra, Amrita, and Janice E. Graham, 'Risk, Choice and the "Girl Vaccine": Unpacking Human Papillomavirus (HPV) Immunisation', *Health, Risk & Society*, XIV (2012), pp. 57–69

Reiter, Paul L., N. Brewer, S. Gottlieb et al., 'Parents' Health Beliefs and HPV Vaccination of Their Adolescent Daughters', *Social Science & Medicine*, LXIX (2009), pp. 475–80

INFLUENZA

Barry, John M., *The Great Influenza: The Epic Story of the Greatest Plague in History* (New York and London, 2004)

Bresalier, Michael, 'Uses of a Pandemic: Forging the Identities of Influenza and Virus Research in Interwar Britain', *Social History of Medicine*, XXV (2012), pp. 400–424

Eyler, John M., 'De Kruif's Boast: Vaccine Trials and the Construction of a Virus', *Bulletin of the History of Medicine*, LXXX (2006), pp. 409–38

Kolata, Gina, *Flu: The Story of the Great Influenza Pandemic of 1918 and the Search for the Virus That Caused It* (New York, 1999)

Neustadt, Richard E., and Harvey V. Fineberg, *The Epidemic That Never Was: Policymaking and the Swine Flu Scare* (New York, 1983)

Tognotti, Eugenia, 'Scientific Triumphalism and Learning from Facts: Bacteriology and the Challenge of the "Spanish Flu" of 1918', *Social History of Medicine*, XVI (2003), pp. 97–110

MALARIA

Desowitz, Robert S., *The Malaria Capers: Tales of Parasites and People* (New York and London, 1991)

Geissler, P. Wenzel, A. Kelly, B. Imoukhuede and R. Pool, '"He Is Now Like a Brother, I Can Even Give Him Some Blood": Relational Ethics and Material Exchanges in a Malaria Vaccine Trial Community in the Gambia', *Social Science & Medicine*, LXVII (2008), pp. 696–707

Packard, Randall, *The Making of a Tropical Disease: A Short History of Malaria* (Baltimore, MD, 2007)

MEASLES, MUMPS AND RUBELLA

Blume, Stuart, and Janneke Tump, 'Evidence and Policymaking:
     The Introduction of MMR Vaccine in the Netherlands', *Social Science
     & Medicine*, LXXI (2010), pp. 1049–55
Galazka, A. M., S. E. Robertson and A. Kraigher, 'Mumps and Mumps
     Vaccine: A Global Review', *Bulletin of the World Health Organization*,
     LXXVII (1999), pp. 3–14
Hendriks, Jan, and Stuart Blume, 'Measles Vaccination before the Measles–
     Mumps–Rubella Vaccine', *American Journal of Public Health*, CIII/8
     (2013), pp. 1393–401
Horstmann, Dorothy M., 'Controlling Rubella: Problems and Perspectives',
     Annals of Internal Medicine, LXXXIII (1975), pp. 412–17
Horton, Richard, MMR *Science and Fiction: Exploring the Vaccine Crisis*
     (London, 2004)
Knox, E. G., 'Strategy for Rubella Vaccination', *International Journal of
     Epidemiology*, IX (1980), pp. 13–23
Vyse, A. J., N. J. Gay et al., 'Evolution of Surveillance of Measles, Mumps,
     and Rubella in England and Wales: Providing the Platform for
     Evidence-based Vaccination Policy', *Epidemiologic Reviews*, XXIV
     (2002), pp. 125–36

POLIO

Blume, Stuart, 'Lock in, the State and Vaccine Development:
     Lessons from the History of the Polio Vaccines', *Research Policy*,
     XXXIV (2005), pp. 159–73
Fairchild, A. L., 'The Polio Narratives: Dialogues with FDR', *Bulletin of the
     History of Medicine*, LXXV (2001), pp. 488–534
Gould, Tony, *A Summer Plague: Polio and its Survivors* (New Haven, CT,
     and London, 1995)
Lindner, Ulrike, and Stuart Blume, 'Vaccine Innovation and Adoption:
     Polio Vaccines in the UK, the Netherlands and (West) Germany,
     1955–65', *Medical History*, I (2006), pp. 425–46
Oshinsky, David, *Polio: An American Story* (New York and Oxford, 2005)
Paul, John R., *A History of Poliomyelitis* (New Haven, CT, 1971)
Renne, Elisha P., *The Politics of Polio in Northern Nigeria* (Bloomington, IN,
     2010)
Sathyamala, C., O. Mittal, R. Dasgupta and R. Priya, 'Polio Eradication
     Initiative in India: Deconstructing the GPEI', *International Journal
     of Health Services*, XXV (2005), pp. 361–83

SMALLPOX AND ITS ERADICATION

Bhattacharya, Sanjoy, 'Re-devising Jennerian Vaccines? European Technologies, Indian Innovation and the Control of Smallpox in South Asia, 1850–1950', *Social Scientist*, XXVI (1998), pp. 27–66

—, 'Uncertain Advances: A Review of the Final Phases of the Smallpox Eradication Program in India, 1960–1980', *American Journal of Public Health*, XCIV (2004), pp. 1875–83

Fenner, Frank, D. A. Henderson, I. Arita, Z. Jezek and I. D. Ladniyi, *Smallpox and its Eradication* (Geneva, 1988)

Franco-Paredes, Carlos, L. Lammoglia and J. Santos-Preciado, 'The Spanish Royal Philanthropic Expedition to Bring Smallpox Vaccination to the New World and Asia in the 19th Century', *Clinical Infectious Diseases*, XLI (2005), pp. 1285–9

Henderson, Donald A., 'Smallpox Eradication: A Cold War Victory', *World Health Forum*, XIX (1998), pp. 113–19

Hennock, E. P., 'Vaccination Policy against Smallpox, 1835–1914: A Comparison of England with Prussia and Imperial Germany', *Social History of Medicine*, XI (1988), pp. 49–71

TUBERCULOSIS AND THE BCG VACCINE

Bonah, Christian, 'Packaging BCG: Standardizing an Anti-tuberculosis Vaccine in Interwar Europe', *Science in Context*, XXI (2008), pp. 279–310

Brimnes, Niels, 'BCG Vaccination and WHO's Global Strategy for Tuberculosis Control, 1948–1983', *Social Science & Medicine*, LXVII (2008), pp. 863–73

—, 'Vikings against Tuberculosis: The International Tuberculosis Campaign in India 1948–51', *Bulletin of the History of Medicine*, LXXXI (2007), pp. 407–3

Bryder, Linda, *Below the Magic Mountain: A Social History of Tuberculosis in Twentieth-century Britain* (Oxford, 1988)

Comstock, George W., 'The International Tuberculosis Campaign: A Pioneering Venture in Mass Vaccination and Research', *Clinical Infectious Diseases*, XIX (1994), pp. 528–40

Gandy, Matthew, and Alimuddin Zumla, 'The Resurgence of Disease: Social and Historical Perspectives on the "New" Tuberculosis', *Social Science & Medicine*, LV (2002), pp. 385–96

Hardy, Anne, 'Reframing Disease: Changing Perceptions of Tuberculosis in England and Wales, 1938–70', *Historical Research*, LXXVI (2003), pp. 535–56

Rosenberg, Clifford, 'The International Politics of Vaccine Testing in Interwar Algiers', *American Historical Review*, CXVII (2012), pp. 671–97

Worboys, Michael, 'From Heredity to Infection: Tuberculosis 1870–1890', in *Heredity and Infection: The History of Disease Transmission*, ed. Jean-Paul Gaudillière and Ilana Löwy (London, 2001), pp. 81–100

WHOOPING COUGH

Blume, Stuart, and Mariska Zanders, 'Vaccine Independence, Local
Competences and Globalisation: Lessons from the History of
Pertussis Vaccines', *Social Science & Medicine*, LXIII (2006), pp. 1825–35
Geier, G. D., and M. Geier, 'The True Story of Pertussis Vaccination:
A Sordid Legacy', *Journal of the History of Medicine*, LVII (2002),
pp. 249–84

ACKNOWLEDGEMENTS

When my late colleague Pieter Streefland invited me to give a talk on 'the development of new vaccines' at a workshop that would form part of the 'Social Science and Immunization Project' he was coordinating, I hesitated. Although I'd been studying the development and introduction of new medical technologies for some years, I knew nothing about vaccines. It didn't take long to discover that there already was a disconcertingly voluminous literature. Nor was it all technical. There were books and articles by historians, economists, health policy analysts, sociologists. A number of leading people in the vaccines field had themselves written thoughtful and reflexive memoires. What could I possibly add that was worth saying and hadn't already been said? Doubtful, I needed to think it over . . . Twenty years ago, when this conversation took place, I could never have imagined that one day I would write this book. I could never have imagined that I'd find the subject so fascinating that I'd still be working on it two decades later. In fact, my fascination with how and by whom vaccines are made, what they are expected to do, and why some people are opposed to them, has only grown over the years. Studying these questions has given me the opportunity of collaborating with some wonderful colleagues. I'd especially like to thank Sidsel Roalkvam, Desmond McNeill, Kristin Sandberg and Jagrati Jani in Norway, Ulrike Lindner and Christine Holmberg in Germany, Judith Justice, Bill Muraskin and Paul Greenough in the United States, Ana-Maria Carrillo in Mexico, Y. Madhavi in India and finally, in the Netherlands, Jan Hendriks, Ingrid Geesink and Anita Hardon. Conversation and collaboration with all of you, at one time or another, has been a privilege and a pleasure. From each of you I have learned something about vaccines, their place in public health and the qualities that make them so important and so intriguing. You won't all agree with everything written here, and for that I offer no apology. Rather I hope it provides the opportunity for further discussion and future collaboration.

Inevitably, over the years I have accumulated intellectual debts to more people than I can possibly name. Influences and borrowings are not always even conscious. So to make it more manageable I'll limit myself to the three years or so in which I've been working on this book. In this time I've been fortunate enough to collaborate on, or at least intensively discuss, a variety of other health-related topics, with many remarkable people. I'm not going to distinguish between friends, colleagues and students, because the categories overlap to so significant an extent. My understanding of medicine and its practice in different specialisms and societies, its place in healthcare more broadly, its limitations and temptations, and my sense of the questions that sympathetic but critical social scientists ought to ask, have profited enormously from all of you. My conversations with each of you have not only been a frequent source of pleasure, but have so often strengthened my determination to continue asking these questions to the best of my ability. I'd like to express my gratitude to Agata Mazzeo, Anja Hiddinga, Beatriz Miranda, Benjamin Meyer Foulkes, Elizabeth Vroom, Heval Özgen, Karina Romo, Katrin Grüber, Lourdes Huiracocha, Maria Fernanda Olarte Sierra, Mia Gisselbaek, Margaret Sleeboom-Faulkner, Nuria Rossell, Radhika Ramasubban, Rob Hagendijk and Selma Tanovic.

Finally, and specifically, I want to thank Ben Hayes at Reaktion for his encouragement; Akiko Kawanami for information on the HPV situation in Japan which I've used in Chapter Seven; Jan Hendriks, Maria Fernanda Olarte-Sierra and David Robbins for commenting on earlier drafts; and Sara Urciuoli for help with production of the index. I hardly need add that any errors of fact, or questionable interpretations, are solely my responsibility.

INDEX